Pocket Guide
for Holistic Nursing

Barbara Montgomery Dossey, RN, PhD, HNC, FAAN
Director
Holistic Nursing Consultan'
Santa Fe, New Me'

Lynn Keegan, RN

Holistic
Port An

Cathie E. Guzzetta, HNC, FAAN
Nursing Research Consultant
Children's Medical Center of Dallas

Director
Holistic Nursing Consultants
Dallas, Texas

JONES AND BARTLETT PUBLISHERS
Sudbury, Massachusetts
BOSTON   TORONTO   LONDON   SINGAPORE

Endorsed by the American Holistic Nurses' Association

World Headquarters

Jones and Bartlett
Publishers
40 Tall Pine Drive
Sudbury, MA 01776
978-443-5000
info@jbpub.com
www.jbpub.com

Jones and Bartlett
Publishers Canada
2406 Nikanna Road
Mississauga, ON
L5C 2W6
CANADA

Jones and Bartlett
Publishers
International
Barb House, Barb
Mews
London W6 7PA
UK

ISBN: 0-7637-4841-2

Production Credits
Acquisitions Editor: Kevin Sullivan
Production Manager: Amy Rose
Associate Production Editor: Tracey Chapman
Editorial Assistant: Amy Sibley
Marketing Manager: Ed McKenna
Associate Marketing Manager: Emily Ekle
Manufacturing Buyer: Amy Bacus
Composition: Auburn Associates, Inc.
Text Design: Paw Print Media
Cover Design: Anne Spencer
Printing and Binding: United Graphics
Cover Printing: United Graphics

Printed in the United States of America
08 07 06 05 04   10 9 8 7 6 5 4 3 2 1

CONTENTS

PREFACE

The *Pocket Guide for Holistic Nursing* was created to provide nurses with a clear and accessible reference to use as they navigate through an explosion of information and an increasing number of challenges in their profession. This guide contains selected and condensed information from *Holistic Nursing: A Handbook for Practice*,[1] and its purpose is three-fold: 1) to expand an understanding of healing and the nurse as an instrument of healing; 2) to explore the unity and relatedness of nurses, clients, and others; and 3) to develop caring–healing interventions to strengthen the whole person.

The *Pocket Guide* is an easy reference for nurses in the art and science of holistic nursing and healing. It also assists nurses in their challenging roles of bringing healing to the forefront of health care and in helping to shape health care reform. We challenge nurses to explore the following three questions:

- What do you know about the meaning of healing?
- What can you do each day to facilitate healing in yourself?
- How can you be an instrument of healing and a nurse healer?

Healing is a lifelong journey into understanding the wholeness of human existence. Along this journey our lives mesh with clients, families, and colleagues, when moments of new meaning and insight emerge in the midst of crisis. Healing occurs when we help clients, families, others, and ourselves embrace what is feared most. It occurs when we seek harmony and balance.

With a new awareness of these interrelationships, healing becomes possible, and the experience of the nurse as an instrument of healing and as a nurse healer becomes actualized. A *nurse healer* is one who facilitates another person's growth toward wholeness (body-mind-spirit), or who assists another with recovery from illness or transition to a peaceful death. Healing is not just curing symptoms. Rather, it is the exquisite blending of technology with caring, love, compassion, and creativity.

As we explore new meanings related to healing in our work and lives, we can weave the many diverse threads of knowledge from nursing as well as from other disciplines. Doing this engenders a more vivid, dynamic, and diverse understanding about the nature of holism, healing, and its implications for nursing. This inner healing allows us to return to our roots of nursing, where healer and healing have always been understood, and to carry Florence Nightingale's vision of health and healing through the new millennium. As she said, "My work is my must." By her shining example, Florence Nightingale invites each of us to find and know our "must" and to explore our own meaning, purpose, and spirituality.[2,3]

This pocket guide is intended for students, clinicians, educators, and researchers who desire to expand their knowledge of holism, healing, and spirituality. This knowledge also can prepare nurses to become certified in holistic nursing, as it presents some of the essential core information of holistic nursing.[4]

The radical changes necessary in health care reform are occurring rapidly. Change has always been the rule in health care. These changes provide us with a greater opportunity to integrate caring and healing into our work, research, and lives. It is up to us to help determine what these new changes will be. We challenge you to capture your essence and to emerge as true healers in this 21st century. Best wishes to you in your healing work and life.

Barbara M. Dossey
Lynn Keegan
Cathie E. Guzzetta

Notes

1. Dossey, B.M., Keegan, L., and Guzzetta, C.E., *Holistic Nursing: A Handbook for Practice*, 4th ed. (Sudbury, MA: Jones and Bartlett, 2005).
2. Dossey, B.M., *Florence Nightingale: Mystic, Visionary, and Healer* (Philadelphia: Lippincott, Williams & Wilkins, 2000).
3. Dossey, B.M., Selanders, L.C., Beck, D.M., and Attewell, A., *Florence Nightingale Today: Healing, Leadership, Global Action* (Washington, DC: Nursesbooks.Org, 2005).
4. Dossey, B.M., *AHNA Core Curriculum for Holistic Nursing* (Sudbury, MA: Jones and Bartlett, 1997).

For more information on the American Holistic Nurses' Association and the AHNA continuing education programs contact:

American Holistic Nurses' Association
P.O. Box 2130 (or) 2733 East Larkin Drive, Suite #2
Flagstaff, AZ 86003-2130
Phone: (800) 278-AHNA or (520) 526-2196
Fax: (520) 426-2752
E-mail: AHNA-flag@flaglink.com
Web Site: www.ahna.org

For information on the holistic nursing certification examination contact:

American Holistic Nurses' Certification Corporation
811 Linden Loop
Cedar Park, TX 78613
Phone: (877) 284-0998
E-mail: ahncc@flash.net
Web Site: www.ahncc.org

CORE VALUE 1

Holistic Philosophy, Theories, and Ethics

CHAPTER 1

Holistic Nursing Practice*

Nurse Healer Objective

- Explore the components of holistic nursing practice.

Definitions

Allopathic/Traditional Therapies: medical, surgery, invasive and noninvasive diagnostic treatment procedures, including medications.

Caring-Healing Interventions: nontraditional therapies that can interface with traditional medical and surgical therapies; may be used as complements to conventional medical and surgical treatments; also called alternative/complementary/integrative therapies or interventions.

Client of Holistic Nursing: an individual, family, group, or community of persons who is engaged in interactions with a holistic nurse in a manner respectful of each client's subjective experience about health, health beliefs, values, sexual orientation, and personal preferences.

Cultural Competence: the ability to deliver health care with knowledge of and sensitivity to cultural factors that influence the health behavior of the person.

Environment: everything that surrounds the person, both the external and the internal (physical, mental, emotional, and spiritual) environment as well as patterns not yet understood.

---

* Condensed from: B.M. Dossey, C.E. Guzzetta, Holistic Nursing Practice, in *Holistic Nursing: A Handbook for Practice*, 4th ed., eds. B.M. Dossey, L. Keegan, C.E. Guzzetta (Sudbury, MA: Jones and Bartlett Publishers, 2005), 5–37.

Healing: the process of bringing together aspects of one's self, body-mind-spirit, at deeper levels of inner knowing leading toward integration and balance with each aspect having equal importance and value; can lead to more complex levels of personal understanding and meaning; may be synchronous but not synonymous with curing.

Healing Process: a continual journey of changing and evolving of one's self through life; the awareness of patterns that support or are challenges/barriers to health and healing; may be done alone or in a healing community.

Health: the state or process in which the individual (nurse, client, family, group, or community) experiences a sense of well-being, harmony, and unity where subjective experiences about health, health beliefs, and values are honored.

Health Promotion: activities and preventive measures such as immunizations, fitness/exercise programs, breast self exam, appropriate nutrition, relaxation, stress management, social support, prayer, meditation, healing rituals, cultural practices, and promoting environmental health and safety.

Holistic Caring Process: see Chapter 14.

Holistic Communication: a free flow of verbal and non-verbal interchange between and among people and significant beings such as pets, nature, and God/Life Force/Absolute/Transcendent that explores meaning and ideas leading to mutual understanding and growth.

Holistic Nurse: a nurse who recognizes and integrates body-mind-spirit principles and modalities in daily life and clinical practice; one who creates a healing space within herself/himself that allows the nurse to be an instrument of healing for the purpose of helping another feel safe and more in harmony; one who shares authenticity of unconditional presence that helps to remove the barriers to the healing process.

Human Caring Process: the moral state in which the holistic nurse brings her or his whole self into relationship to the whole self of significant beings which reinforces the meaning and experience of oneness and unity.

Intention: the conscious awareness of being in the present moment to help facilitate the healing process; a volitional act of love.

Intuition: see Chapter 14.

Patterns/Challenges/Needs: a person's actual and potential life processes related to health, wellness, disease, or illness which may or may not facilitate well-being.

Person: an individual, client, patient, family member, support person, or community member who has the opportunity to engage in interaction with a holistic nurse.

Person-Centered Care: the condition of trust that is created where holistic care can be given and received; the human caring process in which the holistic nurse gives full attention and intention to the whole self of a person, not merely the current presenting symptoms, illness, crisis, or tasks to be accomplished; reinforcing the person's meaning and experience of oneness and unity.

Presence: the essential state or core in healing; approaching an individual in a way that respects and honors her/his essence; relating in a way that reflects a quality of *being with* and *in collaboration with* rather than *doing to*; entering into a shared experience (or field of consciousness) that promotes healing potentials and an experience of well-being.

Spirituality: a unifying force of a person; the essence of being that permeates all of life and is manifested

in one's being, knowing, and doing; the interconnectedness with self, others, nature, and God/Life
Force/Absolute/Transcendent.

Source: Definitions ©2003 American Holistic Nurses' Association (AHNA).
Permission is given to duplicate this document for teaching purposes by an educational institution. Written consent is required for duplication by an author
or publisher. AHNA, P.O. Box 2130, Flagstaff, AZ 86003-2130; phone (800)
278-2462, fax (928) 526-2752; *www.ahna.org.*

Holism

Natural Systems Theory

Derived primarily from the work of von Bertalanffy,[1] natural
systems theory provides a way of comprehending the interconnectedness of natural structures in the universe (Figure 1–1).
In brief, natural structures vary in size from the level of sub-
atomic particles (i.e., quarks) to the universe, but each pos-
sesses specific characteristics within a structure and is governed
by similar principles of organization. Therefore, a change in

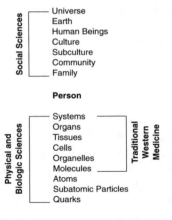

Figure 1–1 Patterns of Natural Systems Components

any one part of the hierarchy affects all other parts. Changes are occurring in all levels simultaneously.

Bio-Psycho-Social-Spiritual Model

The most comprehensive model available to guide mainstream health care is the bio-psycho-social-spiritual model. In this holistic model, all disease has a psychosomatic component, and biologic, psychologic, social, and spiritual factors always contribute to a patient's symptoms, disease, or illness.[2] Each component of the bio-psycho-social-spiritual model is interdependent and interrelated. It is necessary to address all these components to achieve optimal therapeutic results.

Holistic Nursing

Holistic nursing is the most complete way to conceptualize and practice professional nursing. The American Holistic Nurses' Association (AHNA) description of holistic nursing and holism can be obtained from AHNA.[3] (See the Resource List at the end of this chapter for AHNA's address.)

Standards of Holistic Nursing Practice

The AHNA Standards of Holistic Nursing Practice define and establish the scope of holistic practice and describe the level of care expected from a holistic nurse. The framework of the Standards made it possible to develop the *Core Curriculum for Holistic Nursing*,[4] which delineates the fundamental knowledge, competencies, theories, and research for holistic nursing. In turn, the current edition of this book, as well as *Essential Readings in Holistic Nursing*,[5] were developed to expand and augment the knowledge provided in the *Core Curriculum*; all three can be used as major references in teaching holistic nursing as well as in preparing for the AHNA's holistic nursing certification examination. The AHNA's certification examination provides a yardstick by which to measure and confirm that certain individuals are competent to practice holistic nursing as defined by the AHNA. Nurses who pass the examination earn the distinction of certification in holistic nursing and can use the initials HNC (i.e., holistic nurse certified) after their name.

The AHNA *Standards of Holistic Nursing Practice*, revised in 2003, reflect the five core values of holistic nursing, including: core value 1: holistic philosophy, theories, and ethics; core value 2: holistic education and research; core value 3: holistic nurse self-care; core value 4: holistic communication, therapeutic environment, and cultural diversity; core value 5: holistic caring process. The Standards are to be used in conjunction with the American Nurses Association *Nursing: Scope and Standards of Practice* and the standards of the specific specialty in which holistic nurses practice. The Standards describe a diversity of nursing activities in which holistic nurses are engaged. They are used by nurses with expanded practice roles who do not hold graduate degrees, as well as other holistic nurses practicing at the undergraduate level of education.

In 2003 the AHNA created the AHNA *Standards of Advanced Holistic Nursing Practice for Graduate-Prepared Nurses*.[6] The Advanced Standards are based on the same five core values as the basic Standards, but reflect a higher level of performance, proficiency, and expertise. They apply to graduate-level nurses (i.e., those who have a master's or doctoral degree in nursing). AHNA advanced practice certification in holistic nursing soon will be available to graduate-prepared holistic nurses.

Eras of Medicine

Three eras of medicine currently are operational in Western biomedicine.[7] Era I medicine began to take shape in the 1860s. The underlying assumption of this approach is that health and illness are completely physical in nature. The focus is on combining drugs, medical treatments, and technology.

In the 1950s, Era II therapies began to emerge. These therapies reflected the growing awareness that the actions of a person's mind or consciousness exerted important effects on the behavior of the person's physical body. In both Era I and Era II, a person's consciousness is said to be "local" in nature; that is, confined to a specific location in space (the body itself) and in time (the present moment and a single lifetime).

Era III, the newest and most advanced era, originated in science. Consciousness is said to be nonlocal in that it is not bound to individual bodies. The minds of individuals are spread throughout space and time; they are infinite, immortal, omnipresent, and, ultimately, one.

Complementary and Alternative Therapies

Also called unconventional or integrative therapies, complementary and alternative medical (CAM) therapies are defined as a broad set of health care practices (i.e., already available to the public), that are not readily integrated into the dominant health care model because they challenge diverse societal beliefs and practices.[8]

In 1992, the National Institutes of Health (NIH) created the Office of Alternative Medicine (OAM) to evaluate alternative therapies. In 1999, the OAM was raised to the status of a freestanding center and renamed the National Center for Complementary and Alternative Medicine (NCCAM). One of the major missions of the NCCAM is to determine which of these therapies are safe, beneficial, and cost-effective and which are not.

NCCAM has defined five domains, or categories, of CAM.[9] They are 1) Alternative Medical Systems (e.g., traditional Chinese medicine, homeopathic medicine, naturopathic medicine), 2) biologically-based therapies (e.g., macrobiotics, botanical medicines, nutritional supplements), 3) manipulative and body-based methods (e.g., chiropractic medicine, massage therapy, osteopathic manipulation), 4) energy therapies (i.e., therapeutic and healing touch, reiki, Qi gong), and 5) mind-body interventions (e.g., relaxation, imagery, music therapy, prayer). The category of mind-body therapies is predominant in the holistic nursing domain.

In addition, the NCCAM has funded 22 complementary and alternative medicine research centers.[10] Each research center focuses on a specific health condition and is responsible for evaluating the effectiveness and safety of CAM treatments in their specialty area.

The ultimate goal of the CAM therapies movement is not to supplant modern medicine with alternatives, but rather to integrate validated alternative approaches with the best of current conventional medical practices.

Relationship–Centered Care

In 1994, the Pew Health Professions Commission published its report on relationship-centered care. This report serves as a guideline for addressing the bio-psycho-social-spiritual dimensions of individuals in integrating caring, healing, and holism into health care.[11] The guidelines are based on the tenet that relationships and interactions among people constitute the foundation for all therapeutic activities. The three components of relationship-centered care include the patient–practitioner relationship, the community–practitioner relationship, and the practitioner–practitioner relationship. Each of these interrelated relationships involves a unique set of tasks and responsibilities that address self-awareness, knowledge, values, and skills.

Nurse Healer Reflections

- How do I define holism?
- What holistic processes are in need of further development in my personal and professional life?

Notes

1. L. von Bertalanffy, *General Systems Theory* (New York: George Braziller, 1972).
2. B. Dossey, *American Holistic Nurses' Association Core Curriculum for Holistic Nursing* (Sudbury, MA: Jones and Bartlett Publishers, 1997).
3. American Holistic Nurses' Association, *AHNA Standards of Holistic Nursing Practice* (Flagstaff, AZ: AHNA, 2003).
4. B. Dossey, *Core Curriculum for Holistic Nursing*.
5. C.E. Guzzetta, *Essential Readings in Holistic Nursing* (Sudbury, MA: Jones and Bartlett Publishers, 1998).
6. American Holistic Nurses' Association, *AHNA Standards for Advanced Holistic Nursing Practice for Graduate-Prepared Nurses* (AHNA: Flagstaff, AZ, 2003).
7. L. Dossey, *Reinventing Medicine: Beyond Mind-Body To a New Era of Healing* (San Francisco: HarperSanFrancisco, 1999).
8. D.P. Eskinazi, Factors That Shape Alternative Medicine, *Journal of the American Medical Association* 280, no. 18 (1998):1621–1623.
9. Health Information, What is Complementary and Alternative Medicine (CAM)? *http:// nccam.nih.gov.*
10. Research, Research Centers Programs, Funded Research Centers, *http://nccam.nih.gov.*
11. Pew–Fetzer Task Force on Advancing Psychosocial Health Education, *Health Professions Education and Relationship-Centered Care* (San Francisco: Pew Health Professions Commission and the Fetzer Institute, 1994).

Resource List

American Holistic Nurses' Association
P.O. Box 2130
Flagstaff, AZ 86003-2130
Telephone: 1-800-278-2462
Website at *http://www.ahna.org*
For information on holistic certification: *http://www.ahncc.org*

National Center for Complementary and Alternative Medicine Clearinghouse
Website at *http://nccam.nih.gov*

NCCAM Clearinghouse (for questions about the National Center for Complementary and Alternative Medicine Clearinghouse)
P.O. Box 7923
Gaithersburg, MD 20898
Telephone: 1-888-644-6226

CHAPTER 2

Transpersonal Human Caring and Healing*

Nurse Healer Objective
- Explore the components of transpersonal human caring and healing.

Definitions

Healing: the emergence of right relationship at one or more levels of the body-mind-spirit system.[1]

Healing System: a true health care system in which people can receive adequate, nontoxic, and noninvasive assistance in maintaining wellness and in healing for body, mind, and spirit, together with the most sophisticated, aggressive curing technologies available.

Human Caring: the moral ideal of nursing in which the nurse brings his or her whole self into relationship with the whole self of the patient/client, to protect the vulnerability and preserve the humanity and dignity of the one cared for.[2]

Right Relationship: a process of connection among or between parts of the whole that increases energy, coherence, and creativity in the body-mind-spirit system.

Transpersonal: that which transcends the limits and boundaries of individual ego identities and possibilities

---

* Condensed from: J.F. Quinn, Transpersonal Human Caring and Healing, in *Holistic Nursing: A Handbook for Practice,* 4th ed., eds. B.M. Dossey, L. Keegan, C.E. Guzzetta (Sudbury, MA: Jones and Bartlett Publishers, 2005), 41–53.

to include acknowledgment and appreciation of something greater. Transpersonal may refer to consciousness, intrapersonal dynamics, interpersonal relationships, and lived experiences of connection, unity, and oneness with the larger environment, cosmos, or Spirit.

Transpersonal Human Caring

Within the discipline of nursing, there is widespread acceptance of the concept of caring as central to practice. However, there is no widespread consensus as to what caring *is*. Morse and her colleagues reported that five basic conceptualizations, or perspectives, on caring can be identified in the nursing literature: (1) caring as a human trait, (2) caring as a moral imperative or ideal, (3) caring as an affect, (4) caring as an interpersonal relationship, and (5) caring as a therapeutic intervention.[3]

The term *transpersonal human caring* is most often associated with Jean Watson's theory of nursing as the art and science of human caring. Watson defined human caring as the moral ideal of nursing, in which the relationship between the whole self of the nurse and the whole self of the patient/client protects the vulnerability and preserves the humanity and dignity of the patient/client.[4] This emphasis on the whole self—the whole person of both nurse and patient—requires the addition of the term *transpersonal* in Watson's framework and in the discussion of human caring as it relates to holistic nursing practice.

Healing: The Goal of Holistic Nursing

While caring is the context for holistic nursing, healing is the goal. The origin of the word *heal* is the Anglo-Saxon word *haelan*, which means to be or to become whole. Defining what it means to be or become whole is a challenging task. Each holistic nurse should spend some time thinking about what this means to her or him, because a nurse's perspective on wholeness will influence everything that she or he does.

Nurse As Healing Environment

One of the most powerful tools for healing is the presence of the nurse in the patient's environment. In fact, the nurse has the greatest impact of all the elements in the patient's environment. Simply by virtue of the role, a nurse has all the ritual power of the shaman of other cultures. The nurse is guardian of the patient's journey through illness and healing; the keeper and bestower of information, medicines, and treatments; the mediator of the system and the comings and goings of others in the system.

Nurse Healer Reflections

- How do I know when healing is happening in my patients? In myself?

- What gives me true joy and peace in my practice as a holistic nurse, and how can I create more of that?

Notes

1. J. Watson, *Nursing: Human Science and Human Care* (New York: National League for Nursing Press, 1988), 54.
2. J. Quinn, On Healing, Wholeness and the Haelan Effect, *Nursing and Health Care* 10, no. 10 (1989):553–556.
3. J. Morse et al., Concepts of Caring and Caring as a Concept, *Advances in Nursing Science* 13, no. 1 (1990):1–14.
4. Watson, *Nursing: Human Science and Human Care*, 59.

CHAPTER 3

The Art of Holistic Nursing and the Human Health Experience*

Nurse Healer Objective

- Explore the components of the art of holistic nursing and the human health experience.

Definitions

Art of Nursing: the creative mediation and expression of all patterns of knowing in nursing in transformative, aesthetic, and caring holistic nursing actions.

Attitudes: feelings arising out of thoughts, emotions, and behaviors associated with a particular person, idea, or object.

Beliefs: a subset of attitudes that indicate faith in a particular person, idea, or object.

Self-Responsibility: the ability to choose behaviors that are congruent with personal values.

Values: endowment of a particular person, idea, object, or behavior with worth, truth, or beauty.

Values Clarification: a process whereby one becomes more aware of how life values are established and how these values influence one's life.

* Condensed from: H. Gaydos, The Art of Holistic Nursing and the Human Health Experience, in *Holistic Nursing: A Handbook for Practice*, 4th ed., eds. B.M. Dossey, L. Keegan, C.E. Guzzetta (Sudbury, MA: Jones and Bartlett Publishers, 2005), 57–76.

The Art of Holistic Nursing

Nursing is a science, and it is also an art. Those in the field of nursing have made many advances in describing the *science* of nursing. Exactly what constitutes the *art* of nursing is less clear. Interpreting the art of nursing as the "nursing arts" places the emphasis on the proper techniques employed in the tasks of nursing, such as bathing the patient, making the bed, and administering medication. In 1860, however, Florence Nightingale defined the art of nursing as a fine art having to do with the spirit: "Nursing is an art; and if it is to be made an art it requires as exclusive a devotion, as hard a preparation as any painter's or sculptor's work; for what is the having to do with dead canvas or cold marble, compared with having to do with the living body." [1]

Aesthetic Knowing

Carper's landmark study identified the fundamental patterns of knowing in nursing as empirical, ethical, personal, and aesthetic.[2] The aesthetic pattern of knowing is the basis for practice because it mediates and expresses all of the others. Aesthetic knowing is the direct perception of that which is significant in nursing situations.

Aesthetic knowing is said to have two components: "knowledge of the experience toward which the art form is directed and knowledge of the art form itself." [3] Thus, the artful nurse has knowledge of the patient and the human health experience as well as knowledge of nursing.

Creativity

Both science and art are creative and aesthetic. Because holistic nursing is both science and art, the holistic nurse is obligated to uncover or recover, support, and celebrate the creative self. Awakening and cultivating the imaginative mind requires uncovering the heart, opening the mind, letting loose the imagination, creating an environment conducive to creativity, working to master a form, and demonstrating the courage to take risks and be vulnerable.[4] Vulnerability is a key to authenticity, which is requisite because the creative process is a manifestation of the spirit. The physical form of nursing is manifested in acts of caring.

The Cocreative Aesthetic Process[5]

The cocreative aesthetic process may be understood as having four aspects—engagement, mutuality, movement, and new form. These aspects are accurately imagined, not as *parts* of a process but as *facets*, in which each facet is present at all times, but more brilliant when the light of attention is turned on it. These aspects constitute a process that is neither linear nor sequential. Rather, the process has the qualities of skillful improvisation: creativity, spontaneity, integrity, rhythm, and unpredictability. Furthermore, improvisation is unique to the moment and to the people involved—it cannot be recreated or revised. Good improvisation requires excellent intuitive judgment and mature technical skills. Though the process is not linear, it has a discernible beginning and end. It begins with engagement and ends with the creation of a new form. A brief description of each aspect follows:

1. **Engagement** initiates the relationship of one with another and is possible because the participants value each other and the process.
2. **Mutuality** is characterized by the interpenetration of the experience of one person with another. Empathy is essential to this interpenetration. Caring pervades this aspect and is its ethic. The characteristics of the healing relationship are evident in mutuality and include trust, warmth, confidence, credibility, honesty, expectation, courtesy, and respect.[6]

3. **Movement Within and Movement Through** are the two modes of movement experienced in cocreation. Movement within creates rhythm, and movement through creates pattern. Both the rhythm and the pattern are unique to the relationship and to the moment. Movement within (rhythm) is created by a syncopated going back and forth between the self and other. Movement through (pattern) has the characteristic temporal pattern of all human experience: beginning, middle, and end. As the cocreators move through, they go from unknowing to knowing and from unforming to forming. The pattern also refers to the recursive nature of the experience as the cocreators move through and back into engagement and through again from unknowing to knowing and unforming to forming. Unknowing creates space for the other and for new forms. If one or the other of the cocreators already knows, then there is no space to hear or make something new.

4. **New Forms** are cocreated in a process that may be physical, psycho-social-linguistic, intellectual, or transpersonal. Typically, new forms are recognized with relief, gratitude, and sometimes awe. The forms deepen the experience by being the evidence of it and by allowing a reopening of the cocreative experience through reengagement. The process may be recognized by the cocreators as healing, in the sense of revealing or creating a sense of wholeness.

In the cocreative aesthetic process, aesthetics refers to the wholeness of the experience and to its beauty. Nursing is art when the nurse and the other person(s) cocreate aesthetically the circumstances for healing. The cocreative aesthetic process demonstrates that when nursing is art, the experience is both caring and holistic and directed toward *healing with*. As such the cocreative aesthetic process has therapeutic value for both cocreators. It reinvigorates both and creates a transforming bond between the cocreators.

Aspects of the Human Health Experience

Holistic nurses practice their art within the human health experience—the totality of the human condition that contains and reveals the dynamic relationships among health-wellness–disease-illness.[7] Wellness and illness, like health and disease, are often thought of as mutually exclusive and opposite outcomes. In holistic nursing, however, wellness–illness and health–disease are neither mutually exclusive, nor polar opposites, but are part of a process and part of the whole. Events of wellness-illness–health-disease within the human health experience unfold in a dynamic, dialectic relationship that makes it easier to understand that the individual is a changing person in a changing world.

All aspects of the human health experience have both cognitive and affective dimensions. Cognitive dimensions of health–disease can be seen as comprehensible/incomprehensible, manageable/unmanageable, and meaningful/meaningless. Affective themes that appear are joy/despair, acceptance/resentment, power/fear, and anticipation/confusion.

In the practice of artful nursing, the nurse acknowledges the meaning of the health experience for patients. Therefore, developing a more artful practice requires exploration of the dynamics of health-wellness–disease-illness to gain a deeper understanding of the patterns, meanings, and patient responses. Through greater understanding of the range of meanings in general, and the meaning for individual patients in particular, nurses can facilitate the healing process.

Values Clarification and the Human Health Experience

The pioneering work of Raths and colleagues regarding values is widely used in health care settings. This work explores the complexity and differences in values, attitudes, and beliefs.[8] *Values* are affective dispositions about the worth, truth, or beauty of a thought, object, person, or behavior. Values influence decisions, behavior, and nursing practice. *Attitudes* and beliefs are closely related to values. Attitudes are feelings toward a person, object, or idea that include cognitive, affective, and behavioral elements. *Beliefs* are a subclass of attitudes. The cognitive factors involved in beliefs have less to do with facts and more to do with feelings; they represent a personal confidence, or faith, in the validity of some person, object, or idea.

Values clarification is a dynamic process that emphasizes an individual's capacity for intelligent, self-directed behavior. By taking the time to deliberate about values, individuals find their own answers to a variety of questions or concerns. There is no "correct" set of values, because no one set of values is appropriate for everyone. Rather, the process of values clarification establishes a closer fit between what a person *does* and what that person *says*.

The process of values clarification has three steps: choosing, prizing, and acting. In the first step, the person chooses the value freely and willingly, although only after evaluating each alternative and its consequences. The second step is to prize and cherish the decision and to affirm or communicate the choice publicly. The last step in the process is to incorporate the choice into behavior. These steps translate a value into a consistent, repeated behavioral change that confirms the adoption of the particular value. A true value passes through all steps, but not necessarily in the order discussed. Value indicators are beliefs that do not meet all the criteria of true values and tend to be more numerous than actual values. If the individual is motivated to undergo the values clarification process, a value indicator may become a true value.

Nurse Healer Reflections

- When am I artful in my nursing practice?
- How do my values influence my practice?

Notes

1. J. Watson, Introduction: Art and Aesthetics as Passage between the Centuries, in *Art and Aesthetics in Nursing*, eds. J. Watson and P. Chinn (New York: National League for Nursing, 1994), xv.

2. B. Carper, Fundamental Patterns of Knowing in Nursing, Advances *in Nursing Science*, 1 (1978):13–28.

3. K. Gramling, When is Nursing Art? in *The HeART of Nursing: Expressions of the Creative Art in Nursing*, ed. C. Wendler (Indianapolis: Sigma Theta Tau, 2002).

4. L.E. Daniel, Vulnerability as a Key to Authenticity, *Image* 30, no. 2 (1998):191–192.

5. H.L. Gaydos, Illuminated Lives: Cocreated Portraits of Contemporary Women Healers. Doctoral Dissertation, The Union Institute, Cincinnati, OH, 1999.

6. L. Dossey, Samueli Conference on Definitions and Standards in Healing Research: Working Definitions and Terms, *Alternative Therapies* 9, no.3 (2003):A10–A13.

7. L. Jensen and M. Allen, Wellness: The Dialect of Illness, *Image* 25, no. 3 (1993):220–224.

8. L. Raths et al., *Values and Teaching: Working with Values in the Classroom* (Columbus, OH: Charles E. Merrill, 1978).

CHAPTER 4

Nursing Theory in Holistic Nursing Practice*

Nurse Healer Objective

- Explore the components of nursing theory in holistic nursing practice.

Definitions

Concept: an abstract idea or notion.

Conceptual Model: a group of interrelated concepts described to suggest relationships among them.

Framework: a basic structure; the context in which theory is developed; the structure that permits theory to be understood.

Metaparadigm: concepts that identify the domain of a discipline.

Model: a representation of interactions between and among concepts.

Nursing Theory: a framework; a set of interrelated concepts that are testable; a way of seeing the factors that contribute to nursing practice and nursing thought.

World View: a perspective; a way of viewing, perceiving, and interpreting one's experience.

Nursing Theory Defined

A nursing theory is a framework from which professional nurses can think about their work. Theory is a means of interpreting

* Condensed from: N.C. Frisch, Nursing Theory in Holistic Nursing Practice, in *Holistic Nursing: A Handbook for Practice*, 4th ed., eds. B.M. Dossey, L. Keegan, C.E. Guzzetta (Sudbury, MA: Jones and Bartlett Publishers, 2005), 79–90.

one's observations of the world, and is an abstraction of reality. In nursing, there are four basic ideas (or concepts) that are common to all nursing theories—the concepts of nursing, person, health, and environment. These concepts comprise the core content of the discipline—the 'metaparadigm' of nursing.

Since the writings of Florence Nightingale,[1] who is considered to be the first nursing theorist and the founder of "modern secular nursing," nurses have had theories about how to practice nursing. Most of these theories, however, have been developed since the 1960s. Several nurses have put forth their ideas of what nursing is and how nursing care can be delivered to assist clients in achieving health. Many practicing nurses are unaware that the care they give is based on a specific theory. They have learned what nursing is by going to nursing school and working with a set of beliefs or assumptions about nursing and the outcomes of nursing care. Knowledge of several theories gives nurses more choices in thinking about the situations in which they find themselves and their clients. Theory gives nurses tools to guide practice and, because nursing theory is grounded in research, theory provides a scientific basis for nursing care.

The Need for Theory

Whenever the topic of nursing theory comes up, some nurses ask, Why do I need a theory? Isn't being holistic enough? These are very important questions. Nurses committed to holism are kind and compassionate nurses who share a philosophy that emphasizes a "sensitive balance between art and science, analytic and intuitive skills, self-care skills, and the ability to care for patients using the interconnectedness of body, mind, and spirit." [2] Theory suggests, in fact *demands*, that nurses reflect on this philosophy and consider how their practice is working (or not working) to achieve holistic ideals.

The Description of Holistic Nursing developed by the American Holistic Nurses' Association (AHNA) states that "holistic nursing practice draws on knowledge, theories, expertise, intuition, and creativity."[3] All five elements are necessary for the nurse to function in an ideal way: Nursing *knowledge* is essential for the understanding of health and disease states and the various regimens required to achieve health. *Theories* enable one to reflect on practice, and to consider carefully all alternatives of care. *Expertise* is necessary to perform nursing skills, and for the ability to make accurate assessments and decisions about care. *Intuition* is needed to understand the client, and to appreciate the subjective experiences of others. *Creativity* is helpful in solving care problems that seem insurmountable; it provides the nurse with novel ideas and ways of being with clients. Each one of these elements is as important as the others.

Theory Development

Theories develop over time as a theorist defines concepts, suggests relationships between concepts, tests and evaluates the relationships, and modifies the theory based on research findings. When the theorist provides definitions of the concepts and suggests possible relationships, the work is called a "conceptual model." Some writers find the distinction between a theory and a conceptual model irrelevant,[4] and for purposes of this chapter, all works will be called theories. It is important, however, for nurses to understand that theories develop and mature, and that they pass through various stages serving increasingly complex purposes:

1. **Description.** The theory provides definitions of concepts, suggests a way of looking at the world, and provides a framework for describing the phenomena of nursing.
2. **Explanation.** The theory suggests relationships between and among various concepts and gives the nurse a means of explaining observed events.
3. **Prediction.** The theory has research findings that establish clear relationships between aspects of nursing, and the nurse is able to predict outcomes.

4. **Prescription.** The theory is well developed and permits a nurse to prescribe nurse or client actions with confidence in the outcomes.

Most nursing theories are developed to the stage of description and explanation, and theorists and researchers are currently developing nursing theories to the stages of prediction and prescription. Table 4-1 lists the nursing theories more frequently used by holistic nurses, the interventions, and the rationale.

A Word About Definitions of Person

Throughout the years of this debate, the AHNA has been asked to take a stand on the meaning of *whole* in holistic nursing practice. The official AHNA Description of Holistic Nursing states

Table 4-1 Nursing Interventions Most Consistent with Specific Nursing Theories

Theory	Interventions	Rationale
Nightingale's Theory of Environmental Adaptation	Care of the environment to promote order, fresh air, and light	Nursing care to the environment puts the patient in the best condition for nature to act upon him/her and promotes healing.
Roy Adaptation Model	Progressive relaxation Coping enhancement	The nurse evaluates stressors, assists the client to eliminate immediate stress (when possible), and enhances coping strategies in order to adapt to stressors.

Theory	Interventions	Rationale
Modeling and Role Modeling	Guided imagery Hypnotherapy	To "model the client's world," the nurse must focus on timing and pacing of nursing actions. To assist the client to mobilize resources to cope with stress, the modalities of imagery and hypnosis help the client to uncover inherent strengths.
Watson's Theory of Transpersonal Caring	Therapeutic presence Healing presence	To establish a meaningful nurse–client relationship based on caring and the demand for authentic person-to-person exchange, presence is the most important and basic nursing action.
Energy Field Theories	Therapeutic touch (TT) Healing touch modalities	Interventions based on the concepts of the human and environmental energy field are clearly consistent with theories that describe this as their world view.

that holistic nursing is defined primarily as all nursing practice that has the enhancement of healing of the whole person as its goal.[5] The AHNA recognizes that there are two views of holism, and has publicly stated that "holistic nursing responds to both views, believing that the goals of nursing can be achieved within either framework." The important aspect of nursing practice is that the nurse and the client believe that the care received is assisting the client to enhance healing and achieve a state of health. Any nurse who believes that a particular theory is helping to reach the goals mutually set between nurse and client should use the theory and reflect on how the theory's world view changed and assisted nursing practice.

Nurse Healer Reflections

- What definition of the concept of *person* is a good fit with my own view of myself and others?
- Which of the nursing theories described can I use in my practice?
- Which of the nursing theories would be uncomfortable for me to use? Can I openly explore why a particular theory(ies) would be uncomfortable for me to use?
- How will I determine if the theory I am using is acceptable to my clients?
- In what ways am I able and willing to make a contribution to the use and development of nursing theory?

Notes

1. F. Nightingale, *Notes on Nursing* (London: Harrison, 1860).
2. B.M. Dossey, ed., *Core Curriculum for Holistic Nursing* (Sudbury, MA: Jones and Bartlett Publishers, 1997):5–6.
3. American Holistic Nurses' Association (AHNA), *Description of Holistic Nursing* (Flagstaff, AZ: AHNA, 2002).
4. J. George, *Nursing Theories: The Base for Professional Practice*, 5th ed. (Upper Saddle River, NJ: Prentice Hall, 2002).
5. AHNA, *Description of Holistic Nursing*.

CHAPTER 5

Ethics in Our Changing World*

Nurse Healer Objective

- Explore the components of holistic ethics.

Definitions

Being: the state of existing or living.

Consciousness: a state of knowing or awareness.

Ethical Code: a written list of a profession's values and standards of conduct.

Ethics: the study or discipline concerned with judgments of approval or disapproval, rightness or wrongness, goodness or badness, virtue or vice, and desirability or wisdom of actions, dispositions, ends, objects, or states of affairs; disciplined reflection on the moral choices that people make.

Holistic Ethics: the basic underlying concept of the unity and integral wholeness of all people and of all nature, that is identified and pursued by finding unity and wholeness within the self and within humanity. In this framework, acts are not performed for the sake of law, precedent, or social norms, but rather from a desire to do good freely in order to witness, identify, and contribute to unity.

* Condensed from: L. Keegan, Ethics in Our Changing World, in *Holistic Nursing: A Handbook for Practice*, 4th ed., eds. B.M. Dossey, L. Keegan, C.E. Guzzetta (Sudbury, MA: Jones and Bartlett Publishers, 2005), 93–106.

Morals: standards of right and wrong that are learned through socialization.

Nursing Ethics: a code of behavior that influences the way nurses work with those in their care, with one another, and with society.

Personal Ethics: an individual code of thought and behavior that governs each person's actions.

Planetary Ethics: a code of behavior that influences the way in which we individually and collectively interact with the environment and other peoples and animals of the earth.

Values: concepts or ideals that give meaning to life and provide a framework for decisions and actions.

Introduction

Holistic ethics provides guidelines for the development of the healer's spirit and spells out the steps needed to develop the healing attitude. Ethics thus serves as a guide to tap into the wisdom of the cosmos, teaching the individual strategies to release the self to become more participatory in the Greater Self. The participation in the Greater Self forms the linkages between the powers of the cosmos, the healer, and the one to be healed.

Nursing and ethics have been intertwined since the inception of modern nursing. The ethics of nursing comprises both a bedside ethic and a social ethic, as nurses have always concerned themselves in such matters of public policy as urban slums and tenements, war and disaster, and the special needs of the underserved. Recently, the ethics of public policy has also addressed environmental concerns, population issues, human rights, health care delivery, and health promotion. Nurses, both individually and collectively, are directly in the forefront not only of ethical decision making, but also of public policy formation. Many aspects of future health care delivery will be based on the ethical decisions that we make now. Thus, nurses must examine current and future healing activities from ethical perspectives. All of us must strive to understand the concept and application of ethics.

The Nature of Ethical Problems

Because ethical issues consist of diverse values and perspectives, they are extremely complex. Ethical questions arise from all areas of life. The ramifications of the population explosion, euthanasia, genetic engineering, and allocation of resources are only a few examples of a host of controversial ethical issues. Furthermore, four specific recent developments in our society have dramatically increased ethical awareness: (1) advances in medical technology, (2) greater recognition of patients' rights, (3) malpractice cases and court-ordered treatment, and (4) scarcity of resources.[1]

Holistic ethics is a philosophy that couples both reemerging and rapidly evolving concepts of holism and ethics. It involves a basic underlying concept of the unity and integral wholeness of all people, and of all nature, that is identified and pursued by finding unity and wholeness within the self and within humanity. Within the framework of holistic ethics, acts are not performed for the sake of law, precedent, or social norms; they are performed from a desire to do good freely in order to witness, identify, and contribute to unity of the self and of the universe, of which the individual is a part. Encompassing traditional ethical views, the holistic view is characterized by the Eastern monad in the yin–yang mode and the Western concept of masculine and feminine. Holistic ethics is not grounded or judged in the act performed or in the distant consequences of the act, but rather in the conscious evolution of an enlightened individual of raised consciousness who performs the act. The primary concern is the effect of the act on the involved individual and his or her larger self.[2]

Holistic ethics originates in the individual's own character and in the individual's relationship to the universe. In some way, the universe is present totally in each individual; paradoxically, the person is just a small part of that same universe. A holistic view takes into account the relationship of unity of all being.

As a philosophic design for living, holistic ethics is a system for the individual. It appeals to the emotions, senses, aesthetic appreciation, and the inner self as revealed by meditative techniques.

The educative process of holistic ethics is not a matter of memorizing facts or historical perspectives, but is instead a process of developing an attitude of awareness of the sacredness of ourselves and all of nature. It is a process in which there is an expanded view that, for both internal and external transformation, our inner self and the collective greater self have stewardship not only of our bodies, minds, and spirits, but also of our planet and the total universe.[3]

Holistic ethics embraces and strives for the fusion between self and others. In the process, it becomes a cosmic ecology, a flowing with the universal tide of events and a co-creator of celestial harmony. All events and ethical decisions become part of the unfolding of a harmonious order and a realization of potentials. Even tragic events can be analyzed within this harmonious spectrum with full realization of the fusion of relationships. One's own actions can become courageous, truth-full, being-full, beauty-full, assured, detached, and virtuous.[4]

Analysis of Ethical Dilemmas

In order to make decisions appropriately, it is necessary, first, to operate from a set of principles and, second, to have some sort of analytical method to help sort out and classify the elements of the problem. When the cases are institutional and patient care–oriented, there are well-established guidelines for analyzing individual cases in ethics that may be helpful.[5,6] Jonsen and colleagues divided the case analysis process into four components: (1) medical indications, (2) patient preferences, (3) quality of life, and (4) contextual issues. Present in every clinical ethical case, these four topics are necessary for a thorough analysis. The holistic approach adds questions of relationships: Who am I? What is my relationship to others? What other factors are contributing to my decisions? Am I wise and courageous enough to perceive and respect others' differences and honor them as I would honor my own beliefs?

Nurse Healer Reflections

- What new insights do I have about the process of ethics?
- How does ethics fit into my clinical practice?
- Do I have the interest and beginning ability to become involved in an institutional ethics committee?
- What role does ethics play in my day-to-day personal life?
- Am I ready to look at planetary issues from a holistic ethical perspective?

Notes

1. F. Hendrickson and G.L. Deloughery, Ethical Influences on Nursing, in *Issues and Trends in Nursing*, ed. G.L. Deloughery (St. Louis: C.V. Mosby, 1991), 180.
2. L. Keegan and G. Keegan, A Concept of Holistic Ethics for the Health Professional, *Journal of Holistic Nursing* 10, no. 3 (1992):205–217.
3. Keegan and Keegan, A Concept of Holistic Ethics for the Health Professional.
4. Keegan and Keegan, A Concept of Holistic Ethics for the Health Professional.
5. A.R. Jonsen, Case Analysis in Clinical Ethics, *Journal of Clinical Ethics* 1, no. 1 (1990):63–65.
6. A.R. Jonsen et al., *Clinical Ethics: A Practical Approach to Ethical Decisions in Clinical Medicine*, 5th ed. (McGraw Hill/Appleton Lange, 2002).

CORE VALUE 2

Holistic Education and Research

The Psychophysiology of Bodymind Healing*

Nurse Healer Objective

- Explore the components of the psychophysiology of bodymind healing.

Definitions

Autopoiesis: the self-organizing force in living systems.

Chaos: the stable and orderly, but irregular, unpredictable behavior of a complex system.

Cycles: one of the simplest nonlinear behaviors that is periodic and recurrent.

Bodymind: a state of integration that includes body, mind, and spirit.

Limbic-Hypothalamic System: the major anatomic modulating link connecting the brain/mind and the autonomic, endocrine, immune, and neuropeptide systems.

Mind Modulation: the bidirectional interrelationships of thoughts and feelings with neurohormonal messengers of the nervous, endocrine, immune, and neuropeptide systems that support bodymind connections.

Self-Regulation Theory: a person's ability to learn cognitive processing of information to bring involuntary body responses under voluntary control.

---

* Condensed from: G.B. Bartol, N.F. Courts, The Psychophysiology of Bodymind Healing, in *Holistic Nursing: A Handbook for Practice*, 4th ed., eds. B.M. Dossey, L. Keegan, C.E. Guzzetta (Sudbury, MA: Jones and Bartlett Publisher, 2005), 111–133.

New Scientific Understanding of Living Systems

Recent developments in science reveal human beings in a new light. The mechanistic view of the world of Descartes and Newton is giving way to a holistic and ecologic view. The habit of looking at persons from the perspective of the body, mind, or spirit is misleading and creates problems of its own. The body can no longer be considered a machine powered by the mind or spirit, to which health care practitioners apply assorted therapies to effect healing. Rather, humans are now understood to be complex, highly integrative systems that are embedded in and supporting other systems. As we free the scientific imagination and increase our knowledge of laws that are the opposite of mechanistic, such as the concepts of nonlocality and superposition of states in quantum physics, our understanding of living systems will continue to change.[1,2] The term *bodymind* includes the body, mind, and spirit as a unified whole.

Emotions and the Neural Tripwire

The traditional view in neuroscience has been that the sensory organs transmit signals to the thalamus and from there to the sensory process areas of the neocortex,[3] which translates the signals into perceptions and attaches meanings. The signals then move to the limbic system, which sends the appropriate response to the body. This has all changed, however, with the discovery of a separate, smaller bundle of neurons that leads directly from the thalamus to the amygdala (Figure 6–1). Sensory impulses go directly from the sensory organs to the amygdala, allowing for a faster response. The amygdala triggers an emotional response even before the person fully understands what is happening. Taking immediate action, the amygdala sends impulses through the brain to the body. If the stimulus is traumatic, the amygdala responds with extra strength. Emotions are not dispensable, but rather an integral part of the whole.

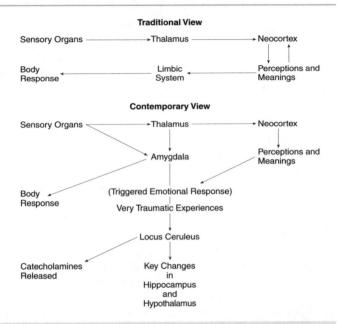

Figure 6-1 Emotions and the Neural Tripwire. Source: Copyright © Genevieve Bartol.

State-Dependent Memory and Recall

What people learn depends on their mood or feelings at the time of the experience.[4] Feelings are integral to human living; they are not just an extravagance or an annoyance. The emotion-carrying molecules, or ligands, which accompany all human activity, bind to cellular receptors and send an informational message to the cell where they can be stored as memories.

Feelings and actions are intertwined. People are more likely to help others when they are in a good mood and more likely to hurt others when they are in a bad mood. Likewise, feelings and memories are intertwined. Thoughts that occur throughout daily routines are repeated patterns of memories and their associative emotional connections. Memories are accompanied by emotions that, in turn, are influenced and affected by the context in which they were acquired. Feelings or mood also play a major role in bodymind healing.

Mind Modulation

Indirect and direct anatomic and biochemical pathways connect the nervous, endocrine, and immune regulatory systems. Communication among these systems is multidirectional, with signal molecules and their receptors regulating the cellular outcomes.[5]

Stress Response

The biochemical functions of the major organ systems are modulated by the mind. Thoughts and feelings are transduced into chemicals (i.e., neurotransmitters, neurohormones, and peptides) that circulate throughout the body and convey messages via cells to various systems within the body. The stress response is a good example of the way in which systems cooperate to protect an individual from harm.

Physiologically, the cascade of changes associated with the stress response appears as tightened muscles; increased heart, respiratory, and metabolic rates; a general sense of foreboding, fear, nervousness, and irritability; and a negative mood. Table 6–1 contains a review of the effects of sympathetic and parasympathetic stimulation.

Pain Response

Pain and suffering are universal and multidimensional experiences. Pain has physical interconnections and physiologic outcomes. Acute and chronic pain differ in several ways. First, acute pain is time-limited, because it occurs with an identifiable problem that generally responds to diagnosis and treatment. Surgery,

Table 6-1 *Effects of Sympathetic and Parasympathetic Stimulation*

Structure	Sympathetic Stimulation	Parasympathetic Stimulation
Pupil of eye	Dilates	Contracts
Ciliary muscle	Relaxes, accommodates for distance vision	Contracts, accommodates for close-up vision
Bronchial tubes	Dilates	Constricts
Heart	Accelerates and strengthens actions	Depresses and slows actions
Stomach muscles	Depresses activity	Increases activity
Glands	Alters secretion	Increases secretion
Liver	Stimulates glycogenolysis	
Visceral muscle of intestine	Depresses peristalsis	Increases peristalsis
Adrenal medulla	Causes secretion of epinephrine	
Sweat glands	Increases activity	Decreases activity
Coronary arteries	Dilates	Constricts
Abdominal and pelvic viscera	Constricts	
Peripheral blood vessels	Constricts	
External genitalia	Constricts blood vessels	Dilates blood vessels, causing erection

Source: Copyright © Genevieve Bartol.

injury, and trauma result in acute pain. Healing of tissue damage usually eliminates the pain. If untreated for 24 hours or longer, however, severe, acute pain can cause neuroplastic changes that lead to "incurable chronic pain syndromes."[6] Neuroplasticity refers to alterations in neuron structure and function resulting from stimulation. Learning and memory produce both chemical and physical neuroplastic changes.

Chronic pain is prolonged, lasting longer than anticipated based on the etiology of the pain. It may be ongoing or may be cyclic, with remissions and exacerbations (such as pain associated with sickle cell anemia, lupus, arthritis, or migraines). Prolonged chronic pain may progress to the point that it becomes the disease or condition. If this occurs, lifestyle changes affecting the person and the family and/or the system of support are common.

PSYCHOSOCIAL PAIN PATHWAYS

Past experiences with pain, emotional state at the time of the pain, and interpretation of the meaning of the pain affect the degree to which the pain is experienced. Both pain recollection and pain anticipation elicit the pain response, just as the recollection of a stressful experience can elicit the stress response (i.e., state-dependent learning).

Pain and suffering are different phenomena. Each can occur without the other, but they can also occur simultaneously. Suffering results when self-image is threatened. Suffering includes spiritual and/or psychosocial anguish,[7] which may be identified through sensitive assessment or by the fact that the pain reaction is greater than expected from the injury. Pain and suffering may appear indistinguishable. The pain response is also shaped by gender, culture, current health states, coping strategies, support, and other issues, such as feelings of control and helplessness.

Nurse Healer Reflections

- Do I attend to my own bodymind communication?
- Do I provide time for self-reflection?
- How do I heighten my awareness of who I am?

Notes

1. F. Capra, *The Web of Life* (New York: Doubleday, 1996), 30.
2. F. Capra, *The Tao of Physics* (Boston: Shambhala, 1999), 67.
3. Pert, *Molecules of Emotion: Why You Feel the Way You Feel*, 350.
4. D. Goleman, *Emotional Intelligence* (New York: Bantam Books, 1995), 6–7, 206–206.
5. J. Shelby and K.L. McCance, Stress and Disease, in *Pathophysiology: The Biologic Basis for Disease in Adults and Children*, eds. K.L. McCance and S.E. Heuther (St. Louis: Mosby, 1998), 298.
6. P. Arnstein, The Neuroplastic Phenomenon: A Physiologic Link between Chronic Pain and Learning, *Journal of Neuroscience Nursing* 29, no. 2 (1997):179–186.
7. E.J. Cassell, Recognizing Suffering, *Hastings Center Report* 21, no. 3 (1991):24–31.

Spirituality and Health*

Nurse Healer Objective

- Explore the components of spiritual caregiving.

Definitions

Spirituality: the essence of our being. It permeates our living in relationships and infuses our unfolding awareness of who and what we are, our purpose in being, and our inner resources. Spirituality is active and expressive. It shapes—and is shaped by—our life journey. Spirituality informs the ways we live and experience life, the ways we encounter mystery, and the ways we relate to all aspects of life. Inherent in the human condition, spirituality is expressed and experienced through living our connectedness with the Sacred Source, the self, others, and nature.

Religion: refers to an organized system of beliefs regarding the cause, purpose, and nature of the universe that is shared by a group of people, and the practices, behaviors, worship, and ritual associated with that system. Religion connects persons through shared beliefs, values, and practices, making clear particular belief systems that are different from other belief systems, thus defining differences between groups of persons.

---

* Condensed from: M.A. Burkhardt, M.G. Nagai-Jacobson, Spirituality and Health, in *Holistic Nursing: A Handbook for Practice*, 4th ed., eds. B.M. Dossey, L. Keegan, C.E. Guzzetta (Sudbury, MA: Jones and Bartlett Publishers, 2005), 137–172.

Spirituality

The term *spirituality* derives from the Latin *spiritus*, meaning breath, and relates to the Greek *pneuma* or breath, which refers to the vital spirit or soul. Spirituality is the essence of who we are and how we are in the world and, like breathing, is integral to our human existence.

Relationship Between Spirituality and Religion

The nursing and health care literature makes it clear that spirituality and religion are not synonymous.[1–3] Spirituality is integral to all persons. As the essence of who we are, spirituality is a manifestation of each person's wholeness and being that is not subject to choice, but simply *is*. Religion per se is not essential to existence. Religion is chosen.

Religion refers to an organized system of beliefs shared by a group of people and the practices related to that system. Ritual, worship, prayer, meditation, style of dress, and dietary observances are examples of such practices.

Elements of Spirituality

Many authors note that spirituality reflects the essence of being; a unifying and animating force; the life principle of each person.[4–6] Spirituality permeates life, shapes our life journey, and is vital to the process of discovering purpose, meaning, and inner strength. Although matters of spirit transcend culture, a person's cultural perspective influences personal expressions of spirituality. Personal values are rooted in and flow from spirituality, and are reflected in a cultural perspective. Spirituality helps to ground one's sense of place and fit in the world. Because it is practical and relevant to daily life, people experience spirituality in the mundane as well as in the profound, the secular as well as the sacred.

CONNECTEDNESS WITH THE SACRED SOURCE

The Sacred Source may be experienced as a person, a presence, or as a mystery that is beyond words. Various cultures, faith traditions, individuals, and groups use names such as Life Force, Source, God, Allah, Lord, Goddess, Absolute, Higher Power, Spirit, Vishnu, Inner Light, Tao, Great Mystery, Tunkasila, The Way, Universal Love, and the One with No Name to refer to that in which we live, and move, and have our being. For this discussion, this Being or Sacred Mystery is referred to as God or the Sacred Source.

CONNECTEDNESS WITH NATURE

Spirituality is frequently expressed and experienced in and through a sense of connectedness with nature, the environment, and the universe.

CONNECTEDNESS WITH OTHERS

Spirituality is known and experienced in and through relationships, with the comfort, support, conflict, and strife that mark those connections. People express and experience spirituality through an appreciation of a common bond with all humanity, and in their particular relationships with others. Spirituality is shaped and nurtured within one's experience of community, beginning with one's family.

CONNECTEDNESS WITH SELF

Spirituality infuses the ever-unfolding awareness of who one is—of self-becoming. The ability to be in the place of awareness that flows from spirit or soul is a pivotal element of connectedness with self. Awareness opens people to the experience of living in the moment, present to their own body-mind-spirit, and allows them to receive all aspects of themselves without judgment. They experience awareness through

Being, the art of stillness and presence with self, others, the Sacred Source, and nature.

Spirituality and the Healing Process

In considering spirituality and healing, it is useful to remember that the words *healing, whole,* and *holy* derive from the same root: Old Saxon *hal,* meaning *whole.* This suggests that, by its nature, healing is a spiritual process that attends to the wholeness of a person.

Spiritual View of Life Issues

Spiritual issues are core "life issues" that often draw people to look into the deepest places in their beings. These issues are not quantifiable and are more authentically expressed as questions, tentative definitions, or as mysteries that cannot be fully explained. They challenge the individual to experience life at its highest heights and deepest depths. Considerations of mystery, love, suffering, hope, forgiveness, grace, peacemaking, and prayer are all inherent in the spiritual domain.

PRAYER

An expression of the spirit, prayer is a deep human instinct that flows from the core of one's being where the longing for and awareness of one's connectedness with the source of life are blended. Prayer represents a longing for communion or communication with God or the Sacred Source.

Forms and expressions of prayer are as varied as the people who pray. Prayer is intrinsic to many religious traditions and rituals. Speaking (sometimes silently), singing, chanting, listening, waiting, moaning, being attuned to what is going on in the present moment, and being silent can all be elements of prayer. Prayer includes petition, intercession, confession, lamentation, adoration, invocation, thanksgiving, being, and showing care and concern for others. Some people incorporate processes and techniques such as relaxation, quieting, breath awareness, focusing, imagery, and visualization into their prayer. Movement such as walking, dancing, or drumming may be expressions of prayer.

Spirituality in Holistic Nursing

Nurturing the Spirit

The way that nurses care for and nurture themselves influences their ability to function effectively in a healing role with another. The *spiritual* path is a *life* path. Attentiveness to one's own spirit is a key component of living in a healing way, and is foundational to integrating spirituality into clinical practice. The many ways nurses nurture their spirits and respond to their spiritual concerns are the same as those that they suggest to their patients. Care of the spirit is a professional nursing responsibility and an intrinsic part of holistic nursing.

Assessing and Investigating Spirituality in Practice and Research

A goal of holistic nursing is to know a person in the fullness and complexity of her or his wholeness. Knowledge obtained about a person through any process of assessment is not an end in itself; rather, it is useful inasmuch as it contributes to understanding and knowing more of the *essence* of the person. Knowledge about a person enables nurses to understand more of who the person is when it is enhanced by the person's perspective of the meaning of such knowledge.

Listening and Intentional Presence

Attentive listening and focused presence are at the heart of caring for the spirit, and they are essential in any approach to spirituality assessment. Good therapeutic communication skills facilitate the exploration of spiritual issues. Broad, open-ended questions are often useful.

Using Story and Metaphor in Spiritual Care

Listening and encouraging people to share their stories can be both assessment and intervention in spiritual care. Stories make it possible to move beyond physical symptoms, diagnoses, and theoretical constructs, which may be similar for any number of patients. Attentiveness to story allows nurses another glimpse into the wholeness and uniqueness of each person and the particular way in which he or she fits into the family and community.

Using Guides and Instruments To Facilitate Spirituality Assessment

Different approaches to assessing spirituality are available to facilitate the integration of spirituality into holistic care.[7] When incorporated into a clinical setting, spirituality assessment guides are a means of gaining a deeper understanding of a person from a holistic perspective. Rather than considering the completion of an instrument to be an end point, nurses can use the questions of an assessment guide as openings or referent points for discussing spirituality with patients and thus come to know and understand them better as unique persons.

The Spiritual Assessment Tool is based on a conceptual analysis of spirituality derived from Burkhardt's critical review of the literature.[8] This instrument poses open-ended, reflective questions that assist nurses in developing awareness of spirituality for themselves and others.

Holistic Caring Process Considerations

Spiritual caregiving requires an understanding of the holistic caring process that is integrative, in which assessment and intervention may well be the same process, and where description may be more useful than labeling. Identification of needs in the area of spirituality does not necessarily indicate pathology or impairment. Research on spirituality and health continues to highlight the importance of describing the human spirit in the language of each person's unique experience and expression, and exploring individual meaning according to the particular person's values. Holistic nurses recognize that spirituality is an important consideration with any health concern, and they use the evolving nursing diagnoses regarding spirituality appropriately. Nurses need to collaborate with clients and their families in determining appropriate outcomes, developing a plan, and organizing overall care to ensure the incorporation of each person's selfhood, values, and world view.

Tending to the Spirit

Care of the spirit, a fundamental aspect of holistic nursing care, takes place in the context of the significant connections in a person's life. The nurse, for a time, enters the client's world and, through intentional presence in this relationship, may facilitate healing. Assessment, diagnosis, planning, and intervening are all experienced within a unique and particular relationship.

Touching

Physical contact through touch in its myriad forms may foster connection. Sensitivity to the meaning of touch for each person is essential in using touch therapeutically. When appropriate, a hand on the shoulder can provide support, a handclasp can convey understanding and presence, an arm around the waist can literally and figuratively give a lift!

Fostering Connectedness

Relationships are a major aspect of spirituality. An awareness and an appreciation of important relationships in the client's life enable the nurse to help strengthen meaningful and supportive bonds. Some family members may need encouragement and guidance in visiting and calling. Clients may need assistance in sharing some aspects of their situation with others—even when they very much want to explain what is happening to them and express their feelings about it. Nurses can remind clients of their network of care and support by recognizing and affirming the support of significant others.

Using Rituals to Nurture the Spirit

Rituals serve as reminders to allow sacred time and space in our lives. Both the ritual behavior and the mindfulness that accompanies it are important aspects of ritual. Achterberg and colleagues described three phases of ritual.[9] The first phase is the *symbolic breaking away* from everyday busyness. The second phase is the *transition phase*, which calls for the identification and focus on areas of life that need attention. The third and final phase, referred to as the *return phase*, is the reentry into everyday life. In essence, ritual gives a person time apart so that he or she may return to the world in a clearer, more centered way. Ritual then can enable nurses to be more intentionally present in healing ways with another.

Developing Centering, Mindfulness, and Awareness

Spiritual disciplines are those practices that cause people to pause in the midst of their activities and busyness to attend to matters of the spirit or soul. The practice of spiritual disciplines requires intention and attention. Eastern and many indigenous traditions around the world emphasize the importance of mindfulness and awareness as disciplines that permeate all of life. Similar to the practice of centering prayer in Judeo-Christian traditions, the mystical path of many traditions calls one to quietness. Making the intentional decision to pause and be mindful of the present moment and all that it holds nurtures the ability to be centered and aware.

Processes of relaxation and imagery facilitate awareness and centering. The practice of spiritual disciplines provides access to a centered space from which the nurse and client can work together, confronting significant life experiences in an environment that is often busy and complex.

Praying and Meditating

Prayer and meditation are spiritual disciplines practiced in many traditions, both cultural and religious. Appreciating the personal nature of these disciplines, the nurse, with respect and sensitivity, can help patients remember or explore ways in which they reach out to and listen for God or the Sacred Source.

Ensuring Opportunities for Rest and Leisure

Holistic nurses try to enhance the patient's conscious awareness of how rest and leisure are, or are not, part of their lives. Such awareness makes those areas available for intentional evaluation, and, if desired, change. Observations and questions may be helpful in the exploration of this aspect of spirituality.

Arts and Spirituality

The arts have a role in the life of the spirit. Many persons find that various forms of artistic endeavor are doors to and expressions of the spirit. An awareness of the breadth of the possibilities of using the arts to enrich the life of the spirit increases the nurse's ability to help the patient use the world of the arts for his or her own journey. The nurse and patient may recognize in books or movies struggles and questions that the patient now confronts, or they may share an appreciation for a special painting, musical piece, or homemade dessert. Providing an atmosphere that, as much as possible, is pleasing to the sensibilities of the patient may promote rest and relaxation. It may also facilitate the use of other interventions, such as imagery.

Nurse Healer Reflections

- In recognizing my wholeness, how would I describe my physical being, my psychologic–emotional being, and my spiritual being?
- What signals spiritual distress in my own life?
- How do I nurture my spirit?
- How would I describe the most significant connections in my life?
- What areas of the spirit need intentional care in my own life?

Notes

1. M.A. Burkhardt and M.G. Nagai-Jacobson, *Spirituality: Living Our Connectedness* (Albany, NY: Delmar Thompson Learning, 2002).
2. J.D. Emblen, Religion and Spirituality Defined According to Current Use in Nursing Literature, *Journal of Professional Nursing* 8 (1992):41–47.
3. Burkhardt and Nagai-Jacobson, *Spirituality: Living Our Connectedness*. (Albany, NY: Delmar Thompson Learning, 2002).
4. Burkhardt, Spirituality: An Analysis of the Concept.
5. J. Walton, Spiritual Relationships: A Concept Analysis, *Journal of Holistic Nursing* 14 (1996):237–250.
6. Burkhardt and Nagai-Jacobson, *Spirituality: Living Our Connectedness*.
7. Burkhardt and Nagai-Jacobson, *Spirituality: Living Our Connectedness*.
8. Burkhardt, Spirituality: An Analysis of the Concept.
9. J. Achterberg et al., *Rituals of Healing: Using Imagery for Health and Wellness* (New York: Bantam Books, 1994).

CHAPTER 8

Energetic Healing*

Nurse Healer Objective

- Explore the components of energetic healing.

Definitions

Aura: an atmosphere; a vague, luminous glow surrounding something. It is an information-containing electromagnetic field and can be likened to the data contained within a computer.

Biophotons: very weak, pulsating ultraviolet (non-visible) light emitted by cells.

Centering: the act of focusing your attention on your heart, resulting in an increase in measurable extra-low frequency magnetic pulses of 0.3–3.0 cycles per second (Hertz), that are emitted by your hands. It can also be called a coherent energetic state.

Chakra: an energy center in the subtle, or energetic, body that is described as a whirling vortex of light.

Consciousness-Created Reality: The quantum theory that proposes that reality exists when a consciousness observes all possible quantum potentialities (wave functions) and selects one.

Energetic: having a capacity for work; active, showing great physical or mental energy.

---

* Condensed from: V.E. Slater, Energetic Healing, in *Holistic Nursing: A Handbook for Practice*, 4th ed., eds. B.M. Dossey, L. Keegan, C.E. Guzzetta (Sudbury, MA: Jones and Bartlett Publishers, 2005), 175–207.

Energetic Healing: The process of using a coherent energy field to induce a change in one's own or another's field.

Hologram: A three-dimensional image produced by an interference pattern of light (as laser light). Each individual part of the interference pattern contains the entire image, which is revealed when the interference pattern is exposed to coherent light of the proper frequency.

Intention: Purpose, aim, or objective. The choice to act in a certain way.

Meridian: parallel pathways that are low voltage electrical conduits. In Eastern philosophies, the meridians are said to conduct chi, or universal energy. The meridians are organized in an electrical mesh that permeates the body and precedes development of vessels and organs.

Psychosynthesis: Assagioli's psychologic theory that proposes a multidimensional human psyche.

Self-referencing Biofeedback: Biofeedback is a technique of learning how to control bodily processes. Self-referencing biofeedback uses internal clues, rather than a machine's response, as a guide. Centering with intention is a self-referencing biofeedback state.

Subtle Energies: Barely noticeable energies from living organisms. Subtle energies are called chi (qi, ki), prana, etheric energy, and mana, among other names, and may be related to electrical and magnetic fields associated with organisms.

Introduction

The philosophy underpinning energetic healing is that the soul/mind precedes energy and that energy precedes biology. Radical, yes. It changes everything. If the soul/mind somehow determines the form energy will take, it is ultimately the builder of biology, chemistry, emotions, relationships—

everything a person experiences. The body, mind, emotions, and spirit are integrated; in other words, they are different reflections of the same energy and of the same consciousness, not separate phenomena. This philosophy enables us to chart our own healing, rather than rely just on outside forces to help us heal. Understanding that energy precedes biology offers very personal avenues of healing and health through our energy fields. To do so, we must encounter our conscious, subconscious, unconscious, and long forgotten choices. Those choices and their aftermaths are held in the energy field as information, as energy in-form-ation. Our job is to engage those forms, recognize them and let them go so we can create new, more appropriate forms of energy, new ways of being.

An Overview of Energetic Healing

Energetic healing is a term used to describe healing that alters the subtle flow of energy within and around a person or organism. This subtle field is essential to the health of the organism, and many cultures have developed healing methods using those energies. This energy flow may be electromagnetic and is called by many names, including chi, ki, qi, mana, prana, and etheric. Energetic healing techniques can be classified as laying-on-of-hands, biofield therapy, and subtle energy healing. Other approaches use light, sound, aromas, and flower essences to influence the subtle energy field. The laying-on-of-hands types of energetic healing have three sources of understanding: (1) traditional conceptions of energetic structures and functions, (2) the personal experiences of energetic healers, and (3) physics.

Energetic therapies work with phenomena that are more familiar to physicists than to biologists. Understanding energetic healing requires knowledge of electricity, electromagnetism, and quantum physics. While energetic healers look to physics to explain what they sense, the explanations are only tentative. Physicists rely on experimental results and mathematical formulas to describe phenomena; until a theory is confirmed experimentally, it is a metaphor. At this point, the physics explanations given energetic healing are metaphors because there is limited experimental data and no mathematical support of the energetic structures and processes described by energetic healers. As the research base grows, physicists, engineers, and other scientists will become interested in measuring the phenomena experienced and described by healers and, in time, they will develop mathematical models to explain it.

The basic tools of energetic healing are (1) the person receiving the healing, (2) the healer, and (3) energetic structures. Holistic nurses use energetic healing to help a person heal physical, emotional, mental, and spiritual pain and wounds. Pain relief, decreased depression and anxiety, wound healing, and spiritual growth are only a few of the many benefits of energetic healing treatments. The most profound changes are not immediately noticeable because healing takes time—sometimes years of participating in a personal healing quest. Many adults live their lives with beliefs and fears that developed in childhood. Moving beyond those limitations requires healing energetic structures, understanding the larger picture and deeper meaning within experiences, and developing higher aspects of ourselves.

Although energetic healing appears to be about the technique being used, the person being healed is the most important part of the healing equation. Expert healers have learned to use themselves as instruments to change the energy flow in the client's meridians, chakras, and aura, which are to the human what electrical wiring, software, and data are to a computer. These structures serve several functions. On the physical level, each acts like a common electrical device or phenomenon; at the more abstract level, they conduct, process, or store information. The meridians, chakras, and aura collect, transmit, process, and store physical energy and the information the energy contains. The details and nuances of every experience one has had can be found in this remarkable electromagnetic field. The expert healer can help people encounter their information and heal it.

The Healer

Energetic healers' responsibility is to develop and maintain themselves as instruments of healing. Any instrument must be calibrated for the job at hand. Motoyama's discovery that practiced meditators control the output of their chakras offers insight into how expert energetic healers maintain a healing state. Self-control such as the meditators displayed is a type of self-referencing biofeedback. Biofeedback uses machines to provide feedback for biological control, but self-referencing biofeedback uses one's awareness of internal states for feedback. Energetic healers learn to use heart rate, sense of peace, inner calm, and other personal states as cues to create a lowered, more stable heart rate and a more coherent electromagnetic field.

Conclusion

Energetic healing is the art of healing structures so that the individual can heal physical, emotional, and spiritual pain. Healing is not instantaneous; it occurs gradually. Energetic healing promotes the *process* of healing. It makes the process more efficient, and increases the likelihood of success. The energetic healer assists the process, but does not direct it. Results depend upon a person's choice and the effort they put into their own healing.

Assagioli's dimensions of the psyche offers a model of two levels of self. The Personal self provides a more limited, ego-centric perspective of events, and the Transpersonal Self a wider view. Energetic healing will help a person access the Transpersonal Self more easily, enabling one's reality to be viewed more globally and making spiritual healing more likely.

In addition to subtle energy healing, such as in Healing Touch, Therapeutic Touch, and Reiki, healing modalities include the senses. Sound, light, smell, and touch impact the body, mind, and emotions. The impact can be incidental, traumatic, or healing. Energetic healers learn to use sensory stimulation for their healing effects.

Energetic healing does not stand alone; it is but one of many tools available to holistic nurses. It can help one heal chakras, meridians, auras; physical, emotional, and spiritual pain; and access the higher levels of the psyche. The goal of holistic nursing and energetic healing is the same: an integration of body, mind, emotion, and spirit, which leads to healing, peace, love, and joy within the self. As people change, so must the energy they emit, and this will change their world. Ultimately the person each of us needs to heal the most is ourselves. Most people who begin using energetic therapies soon realize that the energy they are working with is urging them to do their own healing work. Most will move deliberately into additional self-care, such as counseling, meditating, journaling, and/or receiving regular energetic healing treatments.

Nurse Healer Reflections

- How do my meridians contribute to my awareness?

- How do my chakras participate in processing information in my life?

- How easy is it for me to access my Transpersonal Self? How can I improve this? How can I help clients access their Transpersonal Selves?

- How can energetic healing blend with my practice as a holistic nurse? Do I wish to be a practitioner of energetic therapies, a client, refer clients to energetic healers, or all of the above?

Holistic Nursing Research*

Nurse Healer Objective

- Explore the components of holistic nursing research.

Definitions

Heisenberg's Uncertainty Principle: the idea that one cannot look at a physical object without changing it.

Placebo: a medically inert medication, preparation, treatment, technique, or ritual that has no specific effects on the body and is intended to have no therapeutic value.

Qualitative Research: a systematic, subjective form of research that is used to describe life experiences and give them meaning. Qualitative research focuses on understanding the whole, which is consistent with the philosophy of holistic nursing.

Quantitative Research: a systematic, formal, objective form of research in which numerical data are used to obtain information about the world. Quantitative research embodies the principles of the scientific method and is used to describe variables, examine relationships among variables, and determine cause-and-effect interactions between variables.

Reductionism: the approach of breaking down phenomena to their smallest possible parts.

* Condensed from: C.E. Guzzetta, Holistic Nursing Research, in *Holistic Nursing: A Handbook for Practice*, 4th ed., eds. B.M. Dossey, L. Keegan, C.E. Guzzetta (Sudbury, MA: Jones and Bartlett Publishers, 2005), 211–228.

Research: a diligent, systematic inquiry or investigation to validate and refine existing knowledge and generate new knowledge.

Evidence-Based Practice

The current mandate to use the best evidence that directs our clinical decisions and the actions we take is driven by the goal of achieving effective patient outcomes and making a positive difference in the lives of our patients. Two strategies used to accomplish this goal are the processes of research utilization and, more recently, evidence-based practice. Research utilization focuses on using research in practice in a way that resembles how it was done in the original research study.[1] It is used to translate research knowledge into what we do. In contrast, evidence-based practice involves more than just research utilization. It is the careful, deliberate use of the best available evidence for making decisions about patient care.[2] This process uses theory, clinical decision making, clinical judgment, and knowledge of research findings combined with clinical expertise, as well as patient values and preferences within the context of available resources.[3] Evidence-based practice needs to be reflected in clinical policies, procedures, and standards of practice.

Need to Conduct Holistic Research

The holistic care of clients must be based on the results of research for several reasons. Research provides the direction for selecting interventions with proved effectiveness. When we implement interventions that have been proved effective, patient outcomes are improved.

With the creation of the National Center for Complementary and Alternative Medicine (NCCAM) at the National Institutes of Health (NIH), many complementary and alternative medical (CAM) therapies are now undergoing scientific evaluation to determine whether they affect the clinical course and outcomes of an illness and whether they enhance wellness.

To date, NCCAM has funded many studies to evaluate such therapies as acupressure, massage therapy, electrochemical treatment, hypnosis, music therapy, guided imagery, biofeedback, prayer, and administration of antioxidants. In addition, NCCAM has established 22 research centers in CAM to study the effects of such therapies on major health conditions and in various populations. The results of these studies will provide the scientific basis for determining which CAM therapies work, which ones do not, which ones are harmful, and, most important, which ones improve patient outcomes.

Holistic Research Methods

Quantitative Research

Research can be defined as a diligent, systematic inquiry or investigation to validate and refine existing knowledge as well as to generate new knowledge.[4]

Quantitative research is a systematic, formal, objective process in which numerical data are used to obtain information about the world. Embodying the principles of the scientific method, quantitative research involves (1) descriptive research, used to describe phenomena; (2) correlational research, used to examine relationships between and among variables; (3) quasi-experimental research, used to explain relationships, examine causal relationships, and clarify the reasons for events; and (4) experimental research, used to examine cause-and-effect relationships between variables. The quantitative method, however, does not take into account (1) the responses of the whole human being to variables, (2) the characteristics of one individual's pathway to a particular problem, and (3) the unique patterns and interacting variables of one individual.[5]

Qualitative Research

In his general systems theory (see Chapter 1), von Bertalanffy proposed that the study of systems requires an understanding of the whole rather than investigation of its separate parts. Because quantitative methods seek to find answers only to parts of the whole, nurses have looked to alternative philosophies of science and research methods that are compatible with investigating humanistic and holistic phenomena.[6] Termed qualitative research, this approach is a systematic, subjective form of research that is used to describe and promote an understanding of human experiences such as health, caring, loneliness, pain, and comfort. Qualitative methods are used when little information is known about a phenomenon, or in areas that are difficult to measure.[7] Qualitative research focuses on understanding the whole, which is consistent with the philosophy of holistic nursing.

Qualitative and quantitative methods, however, should not be viewed from an either/or perspective. Both methodologies are needed in holistic research because they provide complementary approaches for more fully understanding a particular problem.

Enhancing Holistic Research

Psychophysiologic Outcomes

The various physiologic instruments available to study the effects of holistic and CAM therapies are often used in combination to develop a physiologic profile of observed outcomes. Psychologic and physiologic outcomes should be used in combination and the effects of these outcomes should be correlated as a means of increasing the validity of the findings and discovering bodymind links. Psychologic and physiologic measurements should be combined in developing new psychophysiologic tools.

Multimodal Interventions

Quantitative intervention studies can be approached more holistically by taking into consideration the interactive nature of the patient's body-mind-spirit. Many of the holistic and CAM interventions, when used in combination as a multi-modal intervention, may have a more powerful effect on outcomes than any one intervention used alone. For example, the combination of relaxation techniques and music therapy has been shown to be effective in producing the relaxation response, particularly in anxious patients; a head-to-toe relaxation script is used first to reduce muscle tension, and then soothing music is added to enhance relaxation.[8] In a recent study evaluating the effects of distraction combined with positioning (i.e., child–parent chest-to-chest sitting position) on the pain and distress of small children undergoing venipuncture, it was believed that distraction combined with positioning and parental support would be more effective than either one of these interventions alone.[9]

The Placebo Response

Placebo means "I will please." The term refers to a medically inert preparation or treatment that has no specific effects on the body and is intended to have no therapeutic benefit. Yet, this medically inert substance or treatment can evoke a placebo response, relieving pain or dramatically affecting the patient's symptoms or disease.

The placebo response (also called the general healing response) has been studied for several decades in a variety of patients. It appears that, for more than one-third of clients, and probably for even more, the pharmacologically inert placebo is able to activate bodymind healing mechanisms.[10, 11, 12]

The essence of the placebo response involves positive attitudes and emotions.[13] Many CAM therapies, such as imagery, music therapy, relaxation, and exercise, increase endorphin production.[14] When clients believe that they are doing something to enhance healing, their endorphin levels can rise. Basic nursing interventions such as touching, giving backrubs, teaching, positioning, and distracting all have the potential to raise endorphin levels.

Nurse Healer Reflections

- What is my role in establishing an evidence-based practice?
- How do I feel about the importance of research in advancing holistic nursing practice?
- What is my role in nursing research?
- How can I become more involved in holistic clinical research?

Notes

1. D.F. Polit, C.T. Beck, and B.P. Hungler, *Essentials of Nursing Research: Methods, Appraisal, and Utilization*, 5th ed. (Philadelphia: Lippincott, 2001), 431.
2. D. Sackett, S. Richardson, W. Rosenberg, and R. Haynes, *Evidence-Based Medicine: How to Practice and Teach EBM* (New York: Churchill Livingstone, 1997).
3. J. Barnsteiner and S. Prevost, How to Implement Evidence-Based Practice, *Reflections on Nursing Leadership* 28, no. 2 (2002): 18.
4. Polit and Hungler, *Essentials of Nursing Research*, 4–28.
5. D.F. Bockmon and D.J. Riemen, Qualitative versus Quantitative Nursing Research, *Holistic Nursing Practice* 2, no. 1 (1987): 71–75.
6. M.C. Silva and D. Rothbart, An Analysis of Changing Trends in Philosophies of Science on Nursing Theory Development and Testing, *Advances in Nursing Science* 6, no. 2 (1984):1–13.
7. M. Sandelowski, "To Be of Use:" Enhancing the Utility of Qualitative Research, *Nursing Outlook* 45 (1997):125–132.
8. C.E. Guzzetta, Effects of Relaxation and Music Therapy on Patients in a Coronary Care Unit with Presumptive Acute Myocardial Infarction, *Heart and Lung* 18 (1989):609–616.
9. K. Cavender, M. Goff, E. Hollon, and C.E. Guzzetta, Parents' Positioning and Distracting Children During Venipucture: Effects on Children's Pain, Fear, and Distress, *Journal of Holistic Nursing* 22, no. 1 (2004):32–56.

10. H. Beecher, The Powerful Placebo, *Journal of the American Medical Association* 159 (1955):1602.
11. J. Frank, Mind-Body Relationships in Illness and Healing, *Journal of Internal Academic Preventative Medicine* 2 (1975):46.
12. E. Rossi, *The Psychobiology of Mind-Body Healing* (New York: W.W. Norton, 1993), 15.
13. Rossi, *The Psychobiology of Mind-Body Healing*, 11–22.
14. C.B. Pert, *Molecules of Emotion: Why You Feel the Way You Feel* (New York: Charles Scribner's Sons, 1997).

CORE VALUE 3

Holistic Nurse Self-Care

The Nurse As an Instrument of Healing*

Nurse Healer Objective

- Explore the components of the nurse as an instrument of healing.

Definitions

Centeredness: a fine-tuned sensitivity to life's inner and outer patterns and processes; a state of balance of self that allows optimum levels of attention and presence to the moment.

Graceful Presence: a presence which flows from the embodiment of Divine love; moving mindfully with a kinesthetic awareness of the sacredness of being grace-filled and graceful; a lightness of being; an intentional love-infused presence.

Nurse As an Instrument of Healing: a nurse who offers unconditional presence and helps remove the barriers to the healing process; one who creates the space, enhances the environment, and is present to the phenomenon of the unfolding of healing in another; a practitioner who opens the opportunity for another to feel safe and bring into alignment that which has been painful and out of relationship with the self, others, Creator, and creation.

* Condensed from: M. McKivergin with contributions by A. Quarberg, The Nurse As an Instrument of Healing, in *Holistic Nursing: A Handbook for Practice*, 4th ed., eds. B.M. Dossey, L. Keegan, C.E. Guzzetta (Sudbury, MA: Jones and Bartlett Publishers, 2005), 233–254.

Presence: a multidimensional state of being available in a situation with the wholeness of one's individual being; the relational style and quality of "being with" rather than "doing to."

Healing

Healing does not occur in a vacuum. Life has its challenges and opportunities in which to learn, heal, and grow. An individual's response to each of those moments determines the effect of any given event upon his or her body, mind, spirit, relationships, work, and life. Understanding responses to life's challenges is critical, as people often are faced with decisions that tip the scales between life-giving or self-destructive behaviors.

The process of healing is one in which the nurse exchanges energy, truth, and communication with clients to help those clients attune to their own healing capacities and implement the healthiest response possible for any given situation. The nurse serves as a mirror to the client in helping reflect in a healing way the essence of the challenge and opportunity at hand. Connections are made in which a sensitive, selfless regard for another opens the door for a meaningful relationship. The immense power evoked in the relationship between the nurse and client is instrumental in the therapeutic process of healing.[1] The essence of the healing relationship is the nature of the nurse's presence.

QUALITIES OF PRESENCE

The skill of being present to others evolves as a nurse gains professional experience. The initial focus for a new nurse is developing the adequate skill level to provide safe care through the acquisition and practice of basic skills and techniques. Maturity in the nursing profession increases the sensitivity of recognizing the connection between a person's life and health, as well as the perception of the person's body as metaphor. With each level of understanding, the nurse's attitude shifts from "What can I do?" to "How can I be with the person in this moment in a way that will provide the best possible outcome?"

Five distinguishing features of nursing presence include:

1. Self-giving to another at the moment at hand; being available and at the disposal of another
2. Listening to the other
3. Knowing the privilege in participating in the healing experience
4. Giving of one's self
5. Being with another in a way the other person perceives as full of meaning[2]

The Concept of Grace and Presence

The concept of grace is multifaceted, for there are physical, psychosocial, and spiritual components within its description. The word grace is derived from the Hebrew root meaning "favor," and is defined in the dictionary as "seemingly effortless beauty or charm of movement, form, or proportion; a disposition to be generous or helpful; Divine love and protection bestowed freely on people." Theologians describe grace as "the living will of God"[3] and "the quality of Divine order." Sanctifying grace is defined as "the supernatural quality Divinely infused in the soul of man, to be used to heal the soul, give power to will the good and grant perseverance."

Exploring the connection between the qualities of presence and the attributes of grace, as noted in the various definitions, suggests an expanded description and definition of a healing or therapeutic presence, namely "graceful presence." Graceful presence is defined as a presence that flows from the embodiment of Divine love; moving mindfully with a kinesthetic awareness of the Sacredness of being grace-filled and graceful; a lightness of being; an intentional love-infused presence.[4] Having the awareness of being infused with the Creator's love and offering it unconditionally is the underlying premise in being a "graceful presence."

Nurse Healer Reflections

- How do I understand healing?
- What do I consider healing to be?
- How do I experience grace in my life?

Notes

1. M.J. McKivergin, The Nurse As an Instrument of Healing, in *Core Curriculum for Holistic Nursing*, ed. B.M. Dossey (Gaithersburg, MD: Aspen Publishers, 1997), 17–25.
2. J.G. Paterson and L.T. Zderad, *Humanistic Nursing* (NY: John Wiley & Sons, 1976).
3. J. Hastings, *The Encyclopedia of Religion and Ethics*, vol. V (NY: Charles Scribner's Sons, 1961).
4. A.L. Quarberg, *Graceful Presence: Using Mindfulness Movement for Deepening Divine Connection*, unpublished position paper for Master's of Arts Degree from St. Mary's University (Minneapolis, MN, 2002).

CORE VALUE 4

Holistic Communication, Therapeutic Environment, and Cultural Diversity

CHAPTER 11

Therapeutic Communication: The Art of Helping*

Nurse Healer Objective

- Explore the components of therapeutic communication.

Definitions

Therapeutic Communication: a systematic way of relating to another person that enhances self-discovery and ownership of personal issues; use of specific communication skills that support self-exploration and offer feedback to the client.

Communication

Communication is constantly occurring, whether with words, silence, or behavior; one may or may not be conscious of the communication. Holistic in nature, communication includes many dimensions that influence one's ability to send and receive a message. One's perception and ability to take a message into account can be complex. "Taking into account" is considered to be the most important factor in the process of communication,[1] as a person experiences simultaneous information from radio, television, children talking, and a spouse

---

* Condensed from: S. Scandrett-Hibdon, Therapeutic Communication: The Art of Helping, in *Holistic Nursing: A Handbook for Practice*, 4th ed., eds. B.M. Dossey, L. Keegan, C.E. Guzzetta (Sudbury, MA: Jones and Bartlett Publishers, 2005), 259–272.

requesting something. Communication occurs only when the receiver takes into account a message from one of the sources or senders, when a message "gets through" to the receiver's consciousness. The receiver maintains control over which message will receive attention.

The process of communication is constant. What changes is the understanding of the process. In nursing, models of communication tend to be linear, reflecting a mechanistic approach in which the nurse develops a message to affect the client in a certain way so that the client will adopt a desired behavior, often around a healthier lifestyle. A feedback loop is used. For example, when the nurse asks the client how he or she is feeling, the client's response is carefully attended to and reflected back in order to ensure clear understanding. This reflection is helpful to both the nurse and the client, and offers a way for both parties to agree on a similar meaning. Using this technique, the client usually feels heard and "cared about," which builds rapport between the client and the nurse.

In the counseling field, there is general debate as to the "helpfulness" of helping. Some take the position that "helping is never helpful," while others believe that "helping is always helpful." Evidence exists on both sides, but the general conclusion of most practitioners is that helping can be helpful. Evidence suggests that competent helpers do make a difference. "Helping is not neutral; it is for better or for worse."[2] Becoming a skilled, competent helper through the use of effective communication is imperative if holistic nurses are to make a significant contribution to healing.

Therapeutic Communication

A counseling approach that makes the client's self-discovery the key focus is a therapeutic communication process that builds a positive, supportive relationship that enables the client to explore his or her personal experience and behavior.

The helper must use many personal skills to achieve therapeutic communication. The aspects of self involved in this process include accurate listening skills, personal awareness, solicitation of personal understanding about one's life and life themes, wisdom, knowledge of the change process which is not linear or in stages, and intuitive knowing.[3] Systematic training in and practice of interpersonal skills has been found to enhance the helper's performance in helping, as well as increase self-efficacy and cognitive complexity. Personal development of the helper occurs as one's understanding of their own communication style and others are highlighted.

Another important element of helping is keeping the majority of focus on the client's wholeness rather than on the dysfunctions that he or she presents. This attention to the whole person provides the energetic emphasis for the client to attain the greatest possible growth. In medicine, however, focus on pathology often dominates the energetic exchange.

In ordinary conversation, participants frequently use skills such as active listening, validation, and questioning. Each participant is usually invested in being heard, as well as in sharing his or her own story. The relationship is expected to be equal in that both parties benefit from the interaction. Often, painful feelings are "cut off" or diminished because many people have difficulty handling emotional issues. Advice is often solicited and given. Pleasing and judging each other are usually parts of the process.

In therapeutic communication, the helper's entire focus is on the client. Initially, the helper puts his or her own reactions, feelings, and thoughts aside to affirm and assist in clarifying the client's personal expression and meaning. As the relationship develops, the helper begins to guide the client deeper into areas of behavior or patterns of which the client may not be fully aware, thus affording greater clarity, ownership, and the opportunity for change. In illuminating patterns, the helper uses per-

sonal awareness, such as reactions during the interaction or exploration of deeper feelings, to provide information for the
client. The purpose of these exchanges is to assist the client in
making desired changes in his or her life.

Nurse Healer Reflections

- How can these therapeutic communication skills become a long-term investment in my life?
- In what way would my personal and professional communications change if I incorporated these skills into
  my life?
- While working with others, do I continuously focus on
  their wholeness or do I see mostly their disturbed patterns?

Notes

1. L. Thayer, *Communication and Communication Systems*
   (Homewood, IL: Richard D. Irwin, 1968).
2. G. Egan, *The Skilled Helper* (Pacific Grove, CA: Brooks/Cole,
   2002).
3. E. Torres-Rivera, L.T. Phan, C. Maddux, M.P. Wilbur, and M.T.
   Garrett, Process Versus Content: Integrating Personal Awareness
   and Counseling Skills to Meet the Multicultural Challenge of
   the Twenty-first Century, *Counseling Education & Supervision*,
   Sept. 2001, vol. 41:1.

Building a Healthy Environment*

Nurse Healer Objective
- Explore each step of the holistic caring process when building a healthy environment.

Definitions

Ambience: an environment or its distinct atmosphere; the totality of feeling that one experiences from a particular environment.

Anthropocentrism: the world view that places human beings as the central fact or final aim of the universe.

Chaos Theory: sometimes called the "new science," offers a way of seeing order and pattern where formerly only the random, the erratic, and the unpredictable had been observed.

Ecology: the scientific study of interrelationships between and among organisms, and between them and all aspects, living and nonliving, of their environment.

Ecominnea: the concept of an ecologically sound society.

Environment: everything that surrounds an individual or group of people: physical, social, psychologic, cultural, or spiritual characteristics; external and internal features; animate and inanimate objects; seen and unseen

---

* Condensed from: L. Keegan, Building a Healthy Environment, in *Holistic Nursing: A Handbook for Practice*, 4th ed., eds. B.M. Dossey, L. Keegan, C.E. Guzzetta (Sudbury, MA: Jones and Bartlett Publishers, 2005), 275–303.

vibrations; frequencies and climate; and energy patterns not yet understood.

Environmental Ethics: a division of philosophy concerned with valuing the environment, primarily as it relates to humankind, secondarily as it relates to other creatures and to the land.

Environmental Justice: a sub-branch of ethics examining the innate and relational value among organisms and all aspects of their environment.

Epistemology: the branch of philosophy that addresses the origin, nature, methods, and limits of knowledge.

Ergonomics: the study of and realization of the importance of human factors in engineering.

Personal Space: the area around an individual that should be under the control of that individual, including air, light, temperature, sound, scent, and color.

Restorative Justice: an ethical perception that directs that environmental damages not only be curtailed, but also repaired and recompensed in some meaningful way.

Superfund Sites: hazardous waste landfills or abandoned manufacturing sites, names of which appear on the Environmental Protection Agency's National Priorities List.

Sustainable Future: meet the needs of the present without compromising the needs of future generations.

Toxic Substance: a substance that can cause harm to a person through either short- or long-term exposure, as by (1) inhalation; (2) ingestion into the body in the form of vapors, gases, fumes, dusts, solids, liquids, or mists; or (3) skin absorption.

Holistic Caring Process

Assessment

In preparing to exercise environmental control, assess the following parameters as they apply to the client:

- Personal space for comfort, lighting, noise, ventilation, and privacy
- Environment for people or objects that induce anxiety
- Awareness that environmental concerns affect individual and family coping skills
- Awareness of objects or other environmental factors in the physical space that induce comfort or discomfort
- Environmental concerns, as well as the family's environmental concerns
- Possible environmental fears (e.g., a feeling of claustrophobia from being confined to a hospital intensive care bed or intravenous lines, or a fear of death because the patient in the next bed just died)
- Grief and its relationship to environmental factors (e.g., Is the client in the same home atmosphere in which the spouse just died? Are others around the client sad and depressed? Are the colors in the environment dark and heavy?)
- Personal health maintenance in relation to environmental factors (e.g., Can the client easily reach self-care hygiene items? Are throw rugs anchored? Are sunglasses worn outside to prevent glare?)
- Ability to maintain and manage his or her own home
- Risk of injury associated with factors in the environment
- Activity deficits as a result of environmental factors
- Home environment for its potential impact on effective parenting
- Potential noncompliance because of environmental factors
- Risk of impairment in physical activity because of environmental factors
- Risk of impairment in respiratory function because of environmental factors, such as feather pillows, polluted or stale air, cigarette smoking, known or suspected allergens, or overexertion with chronic respiratory conditions

- Possible sleep deficit because of agents in the environment, such as lighting, noise, overstimulation, overcrowding, or allergenic pillows
- Alterations in thought processes that may be influenced by environmental factors, such as sensory bombardment with noise, lack of sleep, and transient living patterns

Patterns/Challenges/Needs

The patterns/challenges/needs compatible with environmental interventions and related to the 13 domains of Taxonomy II (see Chapter 14) are as follows:

- Potential for ineffective choices
- Altered self-care
- Altered growth and development
- Potential for sensory perceptual alteration
- Impaired environmental interpretational syndrome
- Potential for knowledge deficit
- Altered comfort
- Altered role performance

Outcomes

Exhibit 12–1 guides the nurse in client outcomes, nursing prescriptions, and evaluation for the use of the environment as a nursing intervention.

Therapeutic Care Plan and Implementation

BEFORE THE SESSION

- Become aware of personal thoughts, behaviors, and actions that may contribute to the teaching, counseling, or caring environment.
- Prepare the physical environment for optimal lighting, seating, air quality, and noise control.

Exhibit 12-1 Nursing Interventions: Environment

Client Outcomes	Nursing Prescriptions	Evaluation
The client will demonstrate awareness of environment.	Assist the client in shaping his or her own personal space environment.	The client personalized his or her own environment.
	Assist the client with choices that contribute to a positive, safe environment for those who share his or her personal and community space.	The client monitored and controlled the noise that he or she contributed to the surrounding area.
		The client respected the rights of others by not polluting air, water, and public places with wastes.
		The client did not violate the personal space of others with tobacco smoke.

(continues)

Exhibit 12-1 (continued)

Client Outcomes	Nursing Prescriptions	Evaluation
	Provide the client with information that helps in expanding concern for the concept of a healthy global environment.	The client participated in discussions, committees, or programs to work for a safe global environment.
The client will avoid contact and exposure to toxic substances and/or hazardous materials.	Give the client ideas for how to participate in safety education programs at his or her place of employment.	The client participated in his or her workplace offerings of environmental safety programs.
	Teach the client the importance of not handling unnecessary toxic substances.	The client did not handle unnecessary toxic substances and educated himself or herself about the dangers of hazardous materials.

- Consider your internal environment. Is it calm, centered, and ready to interact with others?
- Clear your mind of other matters or personal encounters in order to be fully present when meeting with the client.

BEGINNING THE SESSION

- Allow the client to express specific environmental concerns.
- Guide the client to consider changes that would improve his or her personal and employment environment.
- Encourage the client to write down areas of concern or improvement.

DURING THE SESSION

- Encourage the client to initiate specific intervention ideas in his or her personal or professional work environment.
- Suggest to clients that they can serve on the environmental control committee at their place of employment or if their agency does not have one, that they volunteer to form one.
- Urge clients to consider the areas of sound (e.g., noise, music, machinery), air (e.g., quality, smell, circulation), and aesthetics (e.g., art, color, design, texture), as well as other topics specific to the overall environment.
- Educate hospitalized clients about the deleterious effects of too much noise.
- Encourage hospitalized clients to limit the time spent watching television and instead listen to their own personal cassette players with headphones.
- Create mechanisms whereby music, imagery, relaxation, color, aromas, and the like can be introduced into the workplace settings.

AT THE END OF THE SESSION

- Be aware that you function as a role model. As such, modulate your voice. Speak audibly, but softly, during the session.
- Help clients learn practical ways to cope with hazards in the environment.
- Work together to write down goals and target dates.
- Give handout material to support established goals.
- Schedule follow-up sessions.

Specific Interventions

Personal Environment.   Strategies to heal the environment abound on both a personal and a professional level. Personally, we begin to modify our own internal environment. The ability to regulate our state of consciousness, thought patterns, and reactive behaviors gives us the power to move smoothly through external crises both at work and at leisure. Approaching a hectic external environment with internal composure and tranquility makes it possible to transform crises into manageable situations. Clean, clear internal environments can influence all the external environments in which we work and live.

As we develop the optimal workplaces and living areas to foster self-actualizing conditions and maximize bodymind responses, we must be aware of the impact of all aspects of the environment on human health.

Workplace Noise.   It is the accumulation of noises that adds up in decibels and adds up to stress. By becoming increasingly sensitive to all potential environmental stressors, the nurse becomes more attuned to the opportunities for specific interventions.

Planetary Consciousness.   Schuster suggested that there is an impetus and underlying reason for our developing environmental consciousness. She noted that we are all hoping to foster and sustain our fullest conscious participation in the ongoing web of interrelationships.[1] Three points emerge as most salient within the context of nursing in general, and holistic practice in particular.

1. It is important to address the nature of being human and, in our Western mode, the pervasive influence of the self–other dichotomy.
2. We must be aware that we have viable choices of how we want to be and how we represent ourselves in the world.
3. An integration of items 1 and 2 develops a personal orientation to all environmental concerns. With such an orientation, we can act from internal conviction and relatedness, rather than from institutional directives.[2]

It is up to each of us to develop an environmental sensitivity in our daily lives and become increasingly cognizant of our opportunities to institute positive change.

Evaluation

Each environmental intervention should be measured. The nurse can evaluate with the client the outcomes established before the implementation of any interventions (see Exhibit 12–1). To evaluate the results further, the nurse can explore the subjective effects of the experience with the client, based on the evaluation questions in Exhibit 12–2. Nurses have always been sensitive to environmental issues. Historically, nurses have been the health care providers primarily concerned with health promotion, sanitation, and improvement in the quality of life for all people. Our technologic society has raised new issues and concerns, ranging from the use of increasingly toxic substances to high-technology machinery. Last year's methods of handling laboratory specimens and chemotherapy preparations, for example, may be outdated next year. Nurses keep abreast of the changing face of the environment

Exhibit 12-2 Evaluating the Client's Subjective Experience with Environmental Concerns

1. Were you aware that noise, lighting, air quality, space allocation, and workplace toxins could be chronic stressors?
2. Are there any of these potential stressors in your environment? If so, can you do anything to reduce or remove them?
3. Do you realize that you can contribute to a healthier planet by virtue of changing elements in your own personal space?
4. Do you have an environmental sensitivity group at your workplace? If one existed, would you like to be a part of it?
5. Do you feel empowered to be the person who initiates change in your work setting?
6. What are some specific things that you would like to do to create a healthier environment in your personal space or work setting?
7. What is your next step (or your plan) to integrate these changes in your life?

in order to equip themselves with the newest strategies to counteract hazards. Future nurses would be well advised to remember and recall some of the basic nursing tenets of yesteryear that are still most relevant today. These interventions include fresh air, control for a comfortable climate, cheerful colors and sights, and noise reduction.

Much of how we relate to and what we do about environmental issues is based on the development of our personal philosophy. We continue to become increasingly aware that each of the small things that we do for or against the environment has short- and long-term ramifications. Nurses want to be alert for ways to contribute to positive environmental changes for their own lives, their clients' lives, and the overall health of the planet. Environmental concerns are important to all of us, and one person's actions can have a ripple effect on many other lives. Nurses can be key agents to ensure that the environment is held sacred, supported, and tended as it supports and gives life to all of the earth's people.

Nurse Healer Reflections

- How does the environment affect my job satisfaction?
- What are the environmental stressors at work and at home?
- What strategies can I incorporate in my environment to be healthier?
- What things can I do to improve my own personal and workplace environment?
- How can I be involved with environmental issues at work and in my community?

Notes

1. E. Schuster, Earth Dwelling, *Holistic Nursing Practice* 6, no. 4 (1992):1–9.
2. Ibid.

Cultural Diversity and Care*

Nurse Healer Objective

- Explore each step of the holistic caring process when providing culturally competent health care with various clients to facilitate the healing process.

Definitions

Acculturation: the process of the adaptation, assimilation, or accommodation of an individual immigrant or immigrant group to a new culture.

Assimilation: the process of integration, or taking as one's own, of a new culture by an individual immigrant or immigrant group.

Culture: "the complex whole, which includes knowledge, belief, art, morals, laws, custom and any other capabilities and habits acquired by man as a member of society." [1]

Culturally Competent Health Care: the ability to deliver health care with knowledge of and sensitivity to cultural factors that influence the health and illness behaviors of an individual client or family.

Ethnicity: designation of a population subgroup sharing a common social and cultural heritage.

Ethnocentrism: a world view that is based to a great extent on the socialization of individuals within their

* Condensed from: J.C. Engebretson and J.A. Headley, Cultural Diversity and Care, in *Holistic Nursing: A Handbook for Practice,* 4th ed., eds. B.M. Dossey, L. Keegan, C.E. Guzzetta (Sudbury, MA: Jones and Bartlett Publishers, 2005), 307–336.

own culture, to the extent that such individuals believe that all others see the world as they do.

Race: a social classification that denotes a biologic or genetically transmitted set of distinguishable physical characteristics.

Stereotyping: consigning cultural attributes to a group of people based on assumptions, opinions, or attitudes.

Xenophobia: an inherent fear or hatred of cultural differences.

Holistic Caring Process

When engaged in the holistic caring process, nurses need to understand concepts that are affected by cultural background. Six phenomena evidenced in all cultural groups have variations that are relevant to the provision of culturally competent nursing assessment and care:[2,3]

1. **Communication.** There are cultural variations in expression of feelings, use of touch, body contact, gestures, and verbal and nonverbal communication. Language shapes experiences and influences perceptions and actions.

2. **Personal space.** Spatial behavior refers to the comfort level related to personal space, the area that surrounds a person's body. Spatial territoriality is the need to have and to control personal space. Cultures vary in the level of proximity to others that is acceptable.

3. **Time.** Cultures vary in their orientation toward time, both social time and clock time. Social time refers to patterns and orientations related to the ordering of social life, whereas clock time represents an objective, ordered approach of viewing time in a linear fashion that infers causality. Some cultures orient around cyclic approaches that attach time to natural events that repeat, such as seasons or migration patterns.

4. **Social organization.** Families, religious groups, kinship groups, workplace groups, and special interest groups are social organizations. Families vary by structure, dynamics, roles, and organizational patterns. Kinship structures and the relative geographic location of family members have cultural implications.

5. **Environmental control.** Different cultures have different perceptions of the ability of an individual to control nature, the environment, and personal relationships. The locus of control may be external (i.e., an event contingent on luck or fate), internal (i.e., an event contingent on one's own behavior or characteristic), or outside (i.e., an event in harmony with nature, as in some Asian cultures).

6. **Biologic variations.** In a pluralistic culture, it is important to determine those factors that are strictly biologic (i.e., genetic) and those that are ethnic adaptations related to living in a particular environment (e.g., availability of certain types of food) or in certain social conditions (e.g., socioeconomic status or lifestyle). Biologic factors to be considered are body size and structure. Nutritional issues, including food preferences, habits and patterns, and deficiencies all have medical implications.

Assessment

Leininger defines a cultural nursing assessment as "a systematic appraisal or examination of individuals, groups, and communities as to their cultural beliefs, values, and practices to determine specific needs and interventions within the cultural context of the people being evaluated."[4] A cultural assessment should be performed during the initial contact with a client; it may be brief, with questions about ethnic background, religion, family patterns, food preferences, and health practices.[5] Data from a brief assessment can be used to determine the need for a

more in-depth assessment that focuses on more specific parameters, such as nutritional patterns, social support networks, and
coping (Exhibit 13–1).[6]

Patterns/Challenges/Needs

In the cultural domain, client's needs typically involve bio-
physical and psychologic disturbances, alterations, impair-
ments, and distresses. These patterns, challenges, and needs
are largely derived from the conceptual areas of normalcy
based on North American culture and heavily influenced by
biomedicine. Examples of patterns, challenges, and needs asso-

---

Exhibit 13-1   Cultural Areas Critical to a Nursing Assessment

- Nutritional patterns
- Exercise and physical activities
- Decision making: how made, who is involved, and why
- Health and healing practices
- Family organization, structure, and role differentiation and
  child care practices
- Social support networks and relationships
- Spiritual beliefs, rituals, and practices
- Cognitive attributive style and personal/ family coping
  approaches
- Demographics and socioeconomic status, employment
  patterns
- Immigration and cultural history
- Communication style and relationship toward authority

Source: From J. Engebretson, "Cultural Diversity and Care" in *Core
Curriculum for Holistic Nursing,* ed. B.M. Dossey (Sudbury, MA: Jones
and Bartlett Publishers, 1997), 114.

ciated with cultural differences related to the 13 domains of
Taxonomy II are as follows (see Chapter 14):

- **Altered or impaired communication related to language differences or communication style.** Even with
  the aid of translators, language and dialect differences
  may exist based on the region in which the client was
  born (e.g., China).
- **Altered or impaired social interaction related to sociocultural dissonance.** Difficulties in relating with members of the health care team may occur when there are
  socioeconomic or educational gaps.
- **Lack of adherence related to incongruent value systems between provider and client.** Clients may be considered noncompliant with follow-up appointments
  when differences in the perception of time are at the
  root of missed or late appointments.
- **Anxiety related to culturally unusual expectations
  for behavior and treatment; fear related to unknown
  environment or customs.** The biomedical health care
  system may be particularly anxiety-provoking for
  clients whose custom is to be cared for in the home during an illness.

Outcomes

Culturally appropriate outcomes would be developed with the
client for each culturally-related pattern, challenge, or need.

Therapeutic Care Plan and Implementation

Knowledge and acceptance of the client's right to alternative
solutions and modalities should be incorporated into the plan
of care so that the plan is mutually designed. Explanatory models must be integrated into the care plan.[7] The focus should be
on the concept of engagement rather than compliance, as the
concept of compliance implies an authoritative relationship in

which the provider is active and in control while the client is in a passive, accepting role.[8] Engebretson and Littleton have developed an interactive model of cultural negotiation that parallels the nursing process.[9]

Three modes of intervention involving clinical decision making incorporate the client's cultural practices:[10]

1. Cultural preservation and/or maintenance refers to professional actions that retain relevant care values in health promotion, restoration, management of disabilities or chronic illness, and death. Nurses using cultural preservation can support those aspects of the client's culture that positively influence his or her health care.

2. Cultural accommodation and/or negotiation refer to professional actions to bridge the gap between the client's culture and biomedicine for beneficial health outcomes. Nurses using cultural accommodation recognize the cultural relevance of a practice and assist the client to integrate it into the planned treatment, even though the cultural practice has no scientific basis for health promotion or disease prevention.

3. Cultural repatterning and/or restructuring refers to professional actions that help a client improve his or her life pattern while respecting cultural values and beliefs. Nurses using cultural repatterning should assist clients to make changes in, but not discard, cultural behaviors that are harmful, negative, or maladaptive to their well-being.

A variety of healing modalities may be used, depending on the illness and cultural preferences. Touch as communication has culturally specific meaning. Gentle touch may be seen as a caring gesture. Many cultures have traditions of laying on of hands.

Foods or herbs may be used for many different purposes with respect to illness. The use of hot or cold foods may remedy an imbalance in the body. Many preparations are used to purify and remove toxins from the body, such as emetics and colonic irrigations. For the treatment of specific illnesses, herbs used in traditional healing have antiseptic and healing properties.

Many cultures approach healing from a spiritual perspective. Rituals and practices to protect one from evil, disease, or danger include the use of amulets, talismans, ritualistic behavior, the avoidance of taboos, exorcism, and purification or cleansing rituals. Rituals may be positive in nature, including those related to spiritual growth, redemption, and life transitions, such as birth or initiations into adulthood.[11] Individuals also may seek healing forces by sacrifice, penance, and pilgrimages.

Evaluation

Together, the nurse, the client, and any member of the extended family or social group whom the client feels is significant should evaluate desired client outcomes. Evaluation must be woven throughout the entire holistic caring process, as it is essential to obtain validation through mutual understanding when there are differences between the cultural backgrounds of nurse and client. It is important to note the purpose of the activity in evaluating its effectiveness. A massage that is given for the purpose of comfort needs to be evaluated on the basis of comfort, for example, not its medical effect on the disease process. Each component of the health care plan and each nursing intervention should be carefully examined to ensure that it is understandable and acceptable to the client, effective for achievement of short- and long-term goals, and appropriately revised as necessary during the evaluation process. Cultural modifications can be made upon careful evaluation.

Nurse Healer Reflections

- What are my values and beliefs regarding health and illness in relationship to models of healing?
- How do I feel when caring for clients whose cultural backgrounds differ from my own?

- What are my biases and attitudes toward clients with various cultural backgrounds?
- How can I determine if I am offering culturally competent care in a holistic manner?

Notes

1. M.M. Andrews and J.S. Boyle, eds., *Transcultural Concepts in Nursing Care*, 4th ed. (Philadelphia: J.B. Lippincott, 2003).
2. Gigar and Davidhizar, *Transcultural Nursing: Assessment and Intervention*.
3. J. Engebretson and J. Headley, Cultural Diversity and Care, in *Holistic Nursing: A Handbook for Practice, 3rd ed.*, eds. B.M. Dossey, L. Keegan, and C.E. Guzzetta (Sudbury, MA: Jones and Bartlett Publishers, 2000):283–310.
4. M.M. Leininger and M.R. McFarland, *Transcultural Nursing: Concepts, Theories, Research and Practices*, 3rd ed. (New York: McGraw-Hill, Medical Publishing Division, 2002).
5. T. Tripp-Reimer et al., Cultural Assessment: Content and Process, *Nursing Outlook* 32 (1984):78–82.
6. B.M. Dossey et al., eds., *Holistic Nursing: A Handbook for Practice*, 2nd ed. (Gaithersburg, MD: Aspen Publishers, 1995).
7. J. Engebretson, A Multiparadigm Approach to Nursing, *Advances in Nursing Science* 20 (1997):22–34.
8. Dossey et al., *Holistic Nursing: A Handbook for Practice*.
9. J. Engebretson and L. Littleton, Cultural Negotiation: A Constructivist-Based Model for Nursing Practice, *Nursing Outlook* 49 (2001):223–230.
10. Leininger and McFarland, *Transcultural Nursing: Concepts, Theories, Research and Practices*.
11. D. Kinsley, *Health, Healing, and Religion: A Cross-Cultural Perspective* (Upper Saddle River, NJ: Prentice-Hall, 1996).

CORE VALUE 5

Holistic Caring Process

CHAPTER 14

The Holistic Caring Process*

Nurse Healer Objective

- Explore the components of the holistic caring process.

Definitions

Holistic Caring Process: a circular process that involves six steps which may occur simultaneously. These steps are assessment, patterns/challenges/needs, outcomes, therapeutic care plan, implementation, and evaluation.

NANDA: North American Nursing Diagnosis Association.

Nursing Interventions Classification (NIC): a standardized comprehensive classification or taxonomy of treatments that nurses perform, including both independent and collaborative, as well as direct and indirect.[1]

Nursing Outcomes Classification (NOC): "a comprehensive taxonomy of patient outcomes influenced by nursing care."[2]

Patterns/Challenges/Needs: a person's actual and potential life processes related to health, wellness, disease, or illness, which may or may not facilitate well-being.

Taxonomy II: a multiaxial classification schema for the organization of the accepted list of NANDA nursing diagnoses based upon functional domains and classes.[3]

---

* Condensed from: P.J. Potter and C.E. Guzzetta, The Holistic Caring Process, in *Holistic Nursing: A Handbook for Practice*, 4th ed., eds. B.M. Dossey, L. Keegan, C.E. Guzzetta (Sudbury, MA: Jones and Bartlett Publishers, 2005), 341–375.

Taxonomy of Nursing Practice—NANDA/NIC/NOC (NNN): an atheoretical taxonomic framework that describes nursing practice by linking nursing diagnoses with nursing interventions and nursing outcomes. The NNN Taxonomy of Nursing Practice is a formalized common taxonomic structure for nursing practice that incorporates the NANDA/NIC/NOC classifications and possibly other languages as well.[4]

Holistic Caring Process

The holistic caring process is an adaptation and expansion of the nursing process that incorporates holistic nursing philosophy. Focused on establishment of health and well-being within the person, the holistic caring process is circular and includes six steps: assessment, patterns/challenges/needs, outcomes, therapeutic care plan, implementation, and evaluation.

Assessment

Holistic nurses assess each person holistically using appropriate conventional and holistic methods while the uniqueness of the person is honored.[5]

Assessment is the information-gathering phase in which the nurse and the person identify health patterns and prioritize the person's health concerns. A continuous process, assessment provides ongoing data for changes that occur over time. Each nurse–person encounter provides new information that helps to explain interrelationships and validates previously collected data and conclusions. A key to a holistic assessment is to appraise the overall pattern of the responses.[6] The client is the primary source and interpreter of the meaning of information obtained by the assessment process.

Patterns/Challenges/Needs

Holistic nurses identify and prioritize each person's actual and potential patterns/challenges/needs and life processes related to health, wellness, disease, or illness, which may or may not facilitate well being.[7]

Within the second step of the holistic caring process, the nurse describes a person's patterns/challenges/needs based on a standardized language that is understandable to nurses, other health care professionals, the managed care provider, and the person receiving nursing care. Nursing diagnoses as delineated by NANDA provide the most universal descriptor language for common patterns identified by nurses giving care.[8] (See Exhibit 14–1 for the Domains of Nursing Diagnosis based on Taxonomy II.)

A nursing diagnosis can be defined as a "clinical judgment about the individual, family, or community responses to actual and potential health problems/life processes. Nursing diagnoses provide the basis for selection of nursing interventions to achieve outcomes for which the nurse is accountable."[9]

THE DIAGNOSTIC STATEMENT

The diagnostic label is a "concise phrase or term which represents a pattern of related cues" that defines the diagnosis in practice. Related factors are those "factors that appear to show some type of patterned relationship with the nursing diagnosis."[10] A nursing diagnosis and related factors are connected by the phrase 'related to,' forming a two-part diagnostic statement, such as "deficient knowledge about acute myocardial infarction related to unfamiliarity with information resources characterized by verbalization of the problem."

MULTIAXIAL STRUCTURE OF NURSING DIAGNOSES

Since its inception, the NANDA taxonomy has evolved to a multiaxial structure with seven axes.[11]

AXIS 1: The *diagnostic concept*, consisting of one or more nouns (e.g., anxiety; caregiver role strain), is the "principal element or fundamental and essential part, the root, of the diagnostic statement."[12] (For a complete list of nursing diag-

Exhibit 14-1   Taxonomy II: Domains of Nursing Diagnosis

Domain 1: Health Promotion

The awareness of well-being or normality of function and the strategies used to maintain control of and enhance that well-being or normality of function

Domain 2: Nutrition

The activities of taking in, assimilating, and using nutrients for the purposes of tissue maintenance, tissue repair, and the production of energy

Domain 3: Elimination

Secretion and excretion of waste products from the body

Domain 4: Activity/Rest

The production, conservation, expenditure, or balance of energy resources

Domain 5: Perception/Cognition

The human information processing system including attention, orientation, sensation, perception, cognition, and communication

Domain 6: Self-Perception

Awareness about the self

Domain 7: Role Relationships

The positive and negative connections or associations between persons or groups of persons and the means by which those connections are demonstrated

Domain 8: Sexuality

Sexual identity, sexual function, and reproduction

Domain 9: Coping/Stress Tolerance

Contending with life events/life processes

Domain 10: Life Principles

Principles underlying conduct, thought, and behavior about acts, customs, or institutions viewed as being true or having intrinsic worth

Domain 11: Safety/Protection

Freedom from danger, physical injury, or immune system damage, preservation from loss, and protection of safety and security

Domain 12: Comfort

Sense of mental, physical, or social well-being or ease

Domain 13: Growth/Development

Age-appropriate increases in physical dimensions, organ systems, and/or attainment of developmental milestones

Source: Reprinted with permission from North American Nursing Diagnosis Association. *Nursing Diagnoses: Definitions and Classification 2003–2004* (Philadelphia: NANDA, 2003).

noses, see Dossey BM, Keegan L, and Guzzetta CE. *AHNA Holistic Nursing: A Handbook for Practice.* 4th edition. Sudbury, MA: Jones and Bartlett, 2005.) **AXIS 2: Time**, "the duration of a period or interval" may be described as acute (less than six months), chronic (greater than six months), intermittent, or continuous.[13] **AXIS 3:** The **unit of care**, the population referred to by the diagnostic concept, may be an individual, family, group, or community. **AXIS 4: Age**, "the length of time or interval during which an individual has existed," ranges from fetus through old-old adult.[14] **AXIS 5: Health Status** reflects "the position or rank on the health continuum of wellness to illness (or death)," accommodating actual, risk, and wellness diagnoses. **AXIS 6:** The **descriptor or modifier** conveys a "judgment that limits or specifies the meaning of the nursing diagnosis." Descriptors modify the diagnostic concept with a judgment about the person's health response. For example, grieving may be anticipatory or it may be dysfunctional. **AXIS 7: Topology** refers to parts/ regions of the body—all tissues, organs, anatomical sites, or structures.

Outcomes

Holistic nurses specify appropriate outcomes for each person's actual or potential patterns/challenges/needs.[15]

An outcome is a direct statement of a nurse–person identified goal to be achieved within a specific time frame. An outcome indicates the maximum level of wellness that is reasonably attainable.[16] After the person's patterns/challenges/needs have been identified, one or more specific and concisely stated outcomes are written for each. Client outcomes direct the plan of care.

The Nursing Outcomes Classification (NOC) developed by the Iowa Outcomes Project at the University of Iowa provides a comprehensive taxonomy of 330 outcomes organized into seven domains and 29 classes.[17] Outcomes describe the expected effect or influence of the intervention upon the person.

Therapeutic Care Plan

Holistic nurses engage each person to mutually create an appropriate plan of care that focuses on health promotion, recovery, restoration, or peaceful dying so that the person is as independent as possible.[18]

During the planning stage, nurses who use the holistic caring process help the person identify ways to repattern his or her behaviors to achieve a healthier state. A nursing intervention has been defined as "any direct care treatment that a nurse performs on behalf of a client."

Efforts are underway to develop a classification of nursing interventions that parallels the classification of nursing diagnoses. The Iowa Intervention Project developed the Nursing Interventions Classification (NIC), which contains an alphabetic list of 486 interventions.[19]

Implementation

Holistic nurses prioritize each person's plan of holistic care and holistic nursing interventions are implemented accordingly.[20]

Nurses who are guided by a holistic framework approach the implementation phase of care with an awareness that (1) people are active participants in their care; (2) nursing care must be performed with purposeful, focused intention; and (3) a person's humanness is an important factor in implementation. During this phase the various persons deemed appropriate—the nurse, the person, the family, or another person or agency—implement the planned strategies.[21]

Evaluation

Holistic nurses evaluate each person's responses to holistic care regularly and systematically and the continuing holistic nature of the healing process is recognized and honored.[22]

Data about the client's bio-psycho-social-spiritual status and responses are collected and recorded throughout the holistic caring process. The information is related to the person's patterns/challenges/needs, the outcome criteria, and the results of the nursing intervention. The nurse, in collaboration with the person during the course of care, may use measures from the NOC to document the effectiveness of the nursing interventions received. The goal of evaluation is to determine if outcomes have been successful and, if so, to what extent.

Nurse Healer Reflections

- How am I guided in my everyday life and work by the holistic caring process?

- How can I systematically begin to apply the holistic caring process in terms of standardized nursing taxonomies for diagnoses, interventions, and outcomes?

Notes

1. J.C. McCloskey and G.M. Bulechek, *Nursing Interventions Classification (NIC)*, 3rd ed. (St. Louis: Mosby, 2000).
2. M. Johnson and M. Maas, The Nursing Outcomes Classification, *Journal of Nursing Care Quality* 12, no. 5 (1998):9–20.
3. North American Nursing Diagnosis Association, *Nursing Diagnoses: Definitions and Classification, 2003–2004* (Philadelphia: NANDA, 2003).
4. Ibid.
5. American Holistic Nurses' Association, AHNA *Standards of Holistic Nursing Practice* (Flagstaff, AZ: AHNA, 2003).
6. B. Dossey et al., Nursing Diagnoses Use and Issues: American Holistic Nurses' Association, in *Classification of Nursing Diagnoses: Proceedings of the Tenth Conference*, eds. R.M. Carroll-Johnson and M. Paquette (Philadelphia: J.B. Lippincott, 1994), 160–166.
7. American Holistic Nurses' Association, AHNA *Standards of Holistic Nursing Practice*.
8. North American Nursing Diagnosis Association, *Nursing Diagnoses: Definition and Classification, 2001–2002* (Philadelphia: NANDA, 1999), 1–7.
9. North American Nursing Diagnosis Association, *Nursing Diagnoses: Definitions and Classification, 1999–2000* (Philadelphia: NANDA, 1999), 149.
10. North American Nursing Diagnosis Association, *Nursing Diagnoses: Definitions and Classification, 1999–2000*, 150.
11. North American Nursing Diagnosis Association, *Nursing Diagnoses: Definitions and Classification, 2003–2004*.
12. Ibid., 222.
13. Ibid.
14. Ibid., 224.
15. American Holistic Nurses' Association, AHNA *Standards of Holistic Nursing Practice*.

16. J.C. McCloskey and G.M. Bulechek, Classification of Nursing Interventions: Implications for Nursing Diagnoses, in *Classification of Nursing Diagnoses: Proceedings of the Tenth Conference*, eds. R.M. Carroll-Johnson and M. Paquette (Philadelphia: J.B. Lippincott, 1994), 116.

17. S. Moorhead, M. Johnson, and M. Maas, eds., *Nursing Outcomes Classification (NOC)*, 3rd ed. (St. Louis: Mosby, 2004, in press).

18. American Holistic Nurses' Association, *AHNA Standards of Holistic Nursing Practice*.

19. J.C. McCloskey and G. M. Bulechek, *Nursing Interventions Classification (NIC)*.

20. American Holistic Nurses' Association, *AHNA Standards of Holistic Nursing Practice*.

21. Engebretson and Littleton, Cultural Negotiation.

22. American Holistic Nurses' Association, *AHNA Standards of Holistic Nursing Practice*.

CHAPTER 15

Holistic Self-Assessments*

Nurse Healer Objective

- Explore the components of holistic self-assessments.

Definitions

Biodance: The endless exchange of all living things with the earth in which all living organisms participate.

Healing: a process of bringing all parts of one's self together at deep levels of inner knowing, leading toward an integration and balance, with each part having equal importance and value; also referred to as self-healing or wholeness.

Healing Awareness: the conscious recognition and focusing of attention on sensations, feelings, conditions, and facts dealing with needs of self or clients.

Nurse Healer: one who facilitates another person's growth and life process toward wholeness (body-mind-spirit connections), or who assists with recovery from illness or transition to peaceful death.

Process: the continual changing and evolution of one's self through life; the reflection of meaning and purpose in living.

Transpersonal Self: the self that transcends personal individual identity and meaning to include purpose, meaning, values, and unification with universal principles.

---

* Condensed from: B.M. Dossey and L. Keegan, Holistic Self-Assessments, in *Holistic Nursing: A Handbook for Practice*, 4th ed., eds. B.M. Dossey, L. Keegan, C.E. Guzzetta (Sudbury, MA: Jones and Bartlett Publishers, 2005), 379–393.

Transpersonal View: the state that occurs with a person's life maturity whereby the sense of self expands.

Circle of Human Potential

The circle is an ancient symbol of wholeness. As seen in Figure 15–1, the circle of human potential has six areas: physical, mental, emotions, relationships, choices, and spirit. All are important parts of the self that are constantly interacting. When any one part becomes incomplete, the entire circle loses its completeness because all parts are necessary to maintain the whole. When people become aware of their strengths and their weaknesses, they begin to move to their highest capabilities. The area of choices is surrounded by inner and outer dotted circles; these represent the idea that the continually evolving spiritual development of people guides what

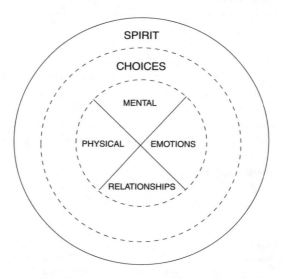

Figure 15–1 Circle of Human Potentials.

they consciously and unconsciously choose. Spirit is placed in the outer circle to show that it transcends all of the other dimensions and helps to maximize our human potentials.

Everyone has the potential—and choice—to tap into this innate healing potential. When we acknowledge our body-mind-spirit relationships, true healing can occur. Times of stress and crisis in our daily routine can block self-healing. Therefore, it is necessary for us to continually assess and reassess our wholeness.

Self-Assessments

In order to maximize our human potentials, it is important to assess each aspect of our being: physical status, mental status, emotions, relationships, choices, and spirit.

Development of Human Potentials

Physical Potential

All humans share the common biologic experiences of birth, gender, growth, aging, and death. Once each person's basic biologic needs for food, shelter, and clothing have been met, there are many ways to seek wholeness of physical potential. Many elements influence physical potential; the major ones are physical awareness of proper nutrition, exercise, relaxation, and balance between work and play. Many people have become obsessed with these elements of the physical potential, but have failed to recognize that they are not separate from—or more important than—the other potentials. Health is more than the absence of pain and symptoms; it is present when there is a balance. As we assess biologic needs, we also must take into consideration our perceptions of these areas. Many illnesses have been documented as stress-related because our consciousness plays a major role in health and physical potential.

Mental Potential

Early in our lives, we have various role models who influence our thoughts, behaviors, and values. As we mature and gain life experience, shifts occur in our thinking, our behavior, and our values. Conflicts develop when we do not take the time to examine our new perceptions and discard old beliefs and values that no longer fit.

Our challenge is to create accurate perceptions of the world through our mental potential. Through both logical and nonlogical mental processes, we become interested in a broad range of subjects and expand our full appreciation of the many great pleasures in life. Not only should we increase our awareness of ways to use both logical and intuitive thought, but also we should increase our skills to create better simultaneous integration of both ways of knowing.

Emotions Potential

Involved in our emotions potential are our willingness to acknowledge the presence of feelings and value them as important, and the ability to express them. Emotional health implies that we have the choice, and freedom, to express love, joy, guilt, fear, and anger. The expression of these emotions can give us immediate feedback about our inner state, which may be crying out for a new way of being.

Emotions are responses to the events in our lives. True healing occurs when we confront both positive and negative intense emotions. Various degrees of chronic anxiety, depression, worry, fear, guilt, anger, denial, or repression result from our failure to confront our emotions. One of the greatest challenges we face is to acknowledge, own, express, and understand our emotions. We are living systems who constantly make exchanges with our environment. All life events affect our emotions and general well-being.

As we become more balanced in living, we allow our humanness to develop. We reach out and ask for human dialogue that is meaningful. Increasing the emotions potential allows spontaneity and a positive, healthy zest for living to emerge. We must be aware of and take responsibility for expression that allows spirit and intuition to flower. It is important to have a consistent harmony between thought processes and emotions, as disharmony causes dissonance.

Relationships Potential

Healthy people live in intricate networks of relationships and are always in search of new, unifying concepts of the universe and social order. Human beings need to explore and develop meaningful relationships. A healthy person simply cannot live in isolation. In a given day, we interact with many people—immediate family, extended family, colleagues at work, neighbors in the community, and numerous people in organizations. Because we spend at least half of our waking hours at work with colleagues, we must support and nourish these relationships. We also must extend our networks to include our nation and planet Earth. Each of us must take an active role in developing local networks of relationships that can have a ripple effect on global concerns.

Choices Potential

People have an enormous capacity for both conscious and unconscious choices in their lives. Conscious choices involve awareness, and skills such as discipline, persistence, goal setting, priorities, action steps, knowledge of options, and recognition of perceptions. We can enhance our awareness, knowledge, and new skills for living and be active participants in daily living, not passive observers who hope that life will be good to us.

Each of us is responsible for assessing our own values and desires. No one else can make decisions for us. When we do not exercise our ability to make choices, the values of others are imposed on us and we never reach our highest potential. Choice involves taking risks. We may make some mistakes along the way, but we also gain experience.

Spirit Potential

Spirit comes from our roots—the universal need to understand the human experience of life on planet Earth. It is the vital element and the driving force in how we live our lives. It impacts every aspect of our life choices and the degree to which we develop our human potentials. Spirit involves the development of our higher self, also referred to as the transpersonal self.

Affirmations

As strong, positive statements acknowledging that something is already so, affirmations can help us change our perceptions and beliefs. If we believe an affirmation to be true, our perceptions selectively reinforce it because we change our self-talk. Our mind is constantly engaged in dialogue with ourselves; in fact, the person we talk to the most in a day is the self. Self-talk even operates in our unconscious through dreams while we sleep. Thus, an important way to influence our unconscious is to focus on positive images and affirmations before we drift to sleep and immediately on awakening. Positive images and affirmations also reinforce those things that have meaning and value. They help us in our spiritual development because they move into the deep layers of the unconscious, become part of our myths, and influence our daily lives.

Nurse Healer Reflections

- What is my process when I assess my circle of human potentials?

- Am I consciously aware of the daily opportunity to manifest my own human potentials?

- What can I do to increase my conscious awareness of fully participating in living?

- How do I feel when I use the word "healer" to describe myself?

CHAPTER 16

Cognitive Therapy*

Nurse Healer Objective

- Explore each step of the holistic caring process when using cognitive therapy with various clients to facilitate the healing process.

Definitions

Cognition: the act or process of knowing.

Cognitive: of or relating to consciousness, or being conscious; pertaining to intellectual activities (such as thinking, reasoning, imagining).

Cognitive Distortions: inaccurate, irrational thoughts; mistakes in thinking.

Cognitive Restructuring: examining and reframing one's interpretation of the meaning of an event.

Cognitive Therapy: a therapeutic approach that addresses the relationships among thoughts, feelings, behaviors, and physiology.

Cognitive Therapy

Cognitive therapy is an important intervention in optimizing the positive links between mind, body, and spirit and in minimizing the negative consequences of adverse interactions.[1,2]

---

* Condensed from: E. Stuart-Shor and C. Wells-Federman, Cognitive Therapy, in *Holistic Nursing: A Handbook for Practice*, 4th ed., eds. B.M. Dossey, L. Keegan, C.E. Guzzetta (Sudbury, MA: Jones and Bartlett Publishers, 2005), 397–425.

Holistic Caring Process

Assessment

In preparing to use cognitive therapy interventions, the nurse assesses the following parameters:

- the client's ability to monitor and appraise inner dialogues and to communicate effectively
- the client's perception of the problem and the degree to which the client wishes to change a thought or behavior
- the client's ability to identify stress warning signals
- the client's readiness for and openness to changing thoughts or behaviors
- the client's level of experience with each of the interventions to be used

Patterns/Challenges/Needs

The following are the patterns/challenges/needs compatible with cognitive therapy.

- Altered verbal/nonverbal communications
- Altered, actual, or potential; Impaired social interaction; social isolation; altered parenting
- Altered coping; ineffective individual and family
- Altered self-concept: disturbance in self-esteem, body image, role performance, personal identity
- Altered thought processes
- Anxiety, fear

Outcomes

- Cognitive therapy helps individuals reappraise, or reevaluate, their thinking. It is often referred to as *cognitive restructuring* because the intent of the intervention is to change or restructure the distortions in thinking patterns that cause stress.

The basic principles of cognitive therapy are:

> — Our thoughts, not external events, create our moods.
> — The thoughts that create stress are usually unrealistic, distorted, and negative.
> — Distorted, illogical thoughts and self-defeating beliefs lead to physiologic changes and painful feelings, such as depression, anxiety, and anger.
> — By changing maladaptive, unrealistic, distorted thoughts, individuals can change how they feel (both physically and emotionally).

• Assist client in the 4-step process of cognitive therapy: awareness automatic thoughts, cognitive distortion, and choosing effective coping.

The goals of cognitive therapy include training clients to

• pinpoint the negative automatic thoughts and silent assumptions that trigger and perpetuate their emotional upsets.
• identify the distortions, irrational beliefs, or *cognitive errors*.
• substitute more realistic, self-enhancing thoughts, which will reduce the stress, symptoms, and/or painful feelings.
• replace self-defeating *silent assumptions* with more reasonable belief systems.
• develop improved social skills, as well as coping, communication, and empathic skills.
• Long-term goals (outcomes) are established prior to therapy, and short-term goals are set prior to each session.
• Goals are set with the client and must be mutually acceptable. A contract may be established to monitor progress and promote adherence.
• A general list of optimal cognitive therapy outcomes includes the following. The client will be able to:

— recognize connections among cognition, emotions, behaviors, and physiology.
— identify physical, psychologic, and behavioral stress warning signals.
— demonstrate the ability to recognize cognitive distortions and examine the evidence for and against key beliefs.
— change the way that he or she thinks (views situations) and try alternative conceptualizations or more rational responses independently.
— report a decrease in arousal, anxiety, fear, depression, or somatic complaints and an elevation in self-esteem after correcting cognitive distortions.

STEP I: AWARENESS

Developing awareness is the first step in a systematic approach to guide clients to a restructuring of their cognitive distortions. Clients are asked to bring to their conscious awareness two things: First, an awareness of how habits of distorted, negative thinking and silent assumptions influence them physically, emotionally, behaviorally, and spiritually. Second, an awareness that a habit pattern (silent assumptions, irrational beliefs, and cognitive distortions) underlies these automatic negative thoughts.

STEP II: AUTOMATIC THOUGHTS

Once the client has been able to identify a stress or a stressful situation, and identify the changes in bodymind that accompany this stress, the next step is to identify the automatic thoughts. These thoughts usually occur automatically in response to a situation. Because these thoughts occur automatically and often are not in the conscious awareness of the individual, they are described as knee-jerk responses. Clients are taught a systematic approach to identifying these self-defeating automatic thoughts.

Exercise to uncover automatic thoughts, feelings, and physical responses.

- **Stop** (break the cycle of escalating, awfulizing thoughts).
- **Take a breath** (release physical tension, promote relaxation).
- **Reflect:**
  — Physically, how do I feel?
  — Emotionally, how do I feel?
  — What are my automatic thoughts (e.g., should, always, ought, never, etc.)?

STEP III: COGNITIVE DISTORTIONS

Once clients have learned to identify stressful situations, their physical, emotional, and behavioral responses to stress, and the automatic thoughts that precipitate the experience, the next step in the process is to teach clients to identify distortions in thinking. Cognitive distortions are illogical ways of thinking that can lead to adverse body-mind-spirit states. The problem is not that these thoughts are wrong or bad, but that people hold the beliefs so strongly. Cognitive distortions are based on beliefs or underlying assumptions that are generally out of proportion to the situation. These beliefs or assumptions are usually long-held, are based on life experience, and often are not in one's conscious awareness.

STEP IV: CHOOSING EFFECTIVE COPING

The final step in the process of cognitive therapy is to help the client restructure or reframe distortions and beliefs and choose a more effective way of responding or coping. To accomplish this, one must recognize that stressful situations have two components, which Ellis termed the *practical problem* and the *emotional hook*. The practical problem is the situation at hand, or the problem that needs to be addressed. The emotional hook is the client's opinion about the problem or the individual(s) who have caused the problem. Quite often people respond to situations as if they can solve the problem by addressing the emotional hook.

Many techniques can be used to help clients effectively problem solve and cope with stressors. Effective coping requires that one attend to both the practical problem and the emotional hook. This sometimes requires two different approaches. Careful thought must be given to each stressful situation in order to choose the most effective coping strategy. The following list suggest a few ways to cope.

Setting Goals

Goal setting is a dynamic process that involves both the client and the nurse at each level. The nurse can facilitate this process by:

- Accumulating a complete bio-psycho-social-spiritual database that is appropriate to the setting and diagnosis.
- Identifying and prioritizing challenges to be addressed.
- Setting mutually agreed-upon short- and long-term goals.
- Helping clients clarify goals.
- Using the 2×50 rule when setting goals. Ask the client to state the goal, then double the amount of time set for accomplishing the goal or reduce its difficulty by 50 percent.
- Establishing a health contract. A health contract is a formal way to enhance goal attainment. It is a way to increase the quality of communication between client and nurse and also can help a client become a more willing participant in self-care. The client's failure to achieve the goals of the contract opens the door to further discussion of the reasons for difficulties with compliance and ways of modifying behavior(s) to achieve a mutually agreed-upon goal.
- A successful contract includes more than simply a list of behavioral goals. Successful attainment of goals de-

pends on skills the client learns during the process of developing the contract. This process provides the opportunity to analyze behaviors in relationship to the environment and to choose strategies that facilitate learning, changing, or maintaining a behavior.

- Contracts may be verbal, but all parties are likely to take written contracts more seriously. If a contract is written, both the client and the nurse should sign it.
- Some clients find the word *contract* threatening or uncomfortable. In this case, the contract may be referred to as an agreement or a statement of mutual goals. In establishing a contract, the nurse assumes the role of facilitator.
- Assisting the client in identifying rewards for achieving a goal. Rewards can enhance goal attainment, but often clients find it difficult to identify appropriate rewards.

Therapeutic Care Plan and Interventions

BEFORE THE SESSION

- Establish a therapeutic relationship by creating a space in which both you and the client feel physically and emotionally safe and comfortable.
- Provide materials for recording cognitive distortions and alternative rational thoughts and statements (e.g., paper and pen, blackboard, preprinted forms).
- Center yourself; clear your mind of personal or professional issues in order to be fully present.
- Establish the long-term goals (outcome) of therapy with the client.

AT THE BEGINNING OF THE SESSION

- Assess the client's level of mood, discomfort, or relaxation.
- Review homework from the previous session, if appropriate. Ask the client to describe any changes that have occurred since the previous session.

DURING THE SESSION

- Determine, with the client, which issues need to be addressed and set short-term goals for the session.
- Listen and guide with focused intention. Provide appropriate feedback, clarification, support, or interpretation.

AT THE END OF THE SESSION

- Have the client identify and verbalize changes that have occurred during the session. Assess progress toward goals.
- Assign homework to be done for the next session.
- Schedule a follow-up session.

Evaluation

Client outcomes that were established prior to initiating cognitive therapy and the client's subjective experiences are used to evaluate progress toward *long-term goals*. To evaluate progress toward *short-term goals*, client outcomes that were established prior to starting the session and the client's subjective experiences are used. Revising and updating goals are a part of each session.

Nurse Healer Reflections

- What are my stress warning signals?
- What are the current stressors in my life?
- Can I pinpoint my negative automatic thoughts and the silent assumptions that trigger and perpetuate my emotional upset?
- Can I use the four-step approach to help reduce my distress and effectively solve problems?
- Is there an affirmation I can create to help me counter self-defeating automatic thoughts and silent assumptions?
- Are my goals realistic?

Notes

1. H. Benson and E. Stuart, *The Wellness Book: A Comprehensive Guide to Maintaining Health and Treating Stress-Related Illness* (New York: Fireside, Simon & Schuster, 1993).
2. E.M. Stuart et al., Spirituality in Health and Healing: A Clinical Program, *Holistic Nursing Practice* 3 (1989):35–36.

CHAPTER 17

Self-Reflection*

Nurse Healer Objective

- Explore each step of the holistic caring process when considering self-reflection.

Definitions

Awareness: alertness, watchfulness, and knowledge about oneself and the environment, including events that take place.

Health: harmony or unity of one's body-mind-spirit within an ever-changing environment.

Identity Status: one of four categories of adolescent identity formation processes.

Self: a principle underlying and organizing subjective experience.

Self-Identity: the process of awareness of who one is and what one's place in the world is.

Self-Reflection: the process of turning awareness inward, communicating with one's inner wisdom for the purpose of healing and well-being.

Holistic Caring Process

Assessment

In preparing to use self-reflection interventions, the nurse assesses the following parameters:

* Condensed from: L. Rew, Self-Reflection, in *Holistic Nursing: A Handbook for Practice*, 4th ed., eds. B.M. Dossey, L. Keegan, C.E. Guzzetta (Sudbury, MA: Jones and Bartlett Publishers, 2005), 429–447.

- **the client's belief system:** Is it congruent with planned interventions?
- **the client's ability to read and write:** If the client cannot read or write, can family members or friends assist with audiotape recordings?
- **the client's experience with similar techniques:** Has the client ever kept a diary or discussed his or her dreams with others?
- **the client's personal goals and motivation for reaching them:** Are they clear to the nurse, and can the nurse respect them if they are different from her own?
- **the client's understanding of the purpose of the intervention:** Does the client understand that the purpose is not to invade his or her privacy, but to enhance self-understanding?

Patterns/Challenges/Needs

The following are the patterns/challenges/needs compatible with the interventions for self-reflection that are related to the 13 domains of Taxonomy II (see Chapter 14):

- Altered communication: impaired verbal communication
- Impaired social interaction; altered family processes; social isolation
- Spiritual distress; disruption of person–environment pattern of the whole
- Impaired adjustment; ineffective family coping; ineffective individual coping
- Activity intolerance: fatigue; sleep pattern disturbance; deficit in diversional activity
- Altered self-concept; body image disturbance; hopelessness; powerlessness
- Altered thought processes
- Anxiety; grieving: anticipatory and dysfunctional

Outcomes

Exhibit 17–1 guides the nurse in client outcomes, nursing prescriptions, and evaluation for the use of self-reflection as a nursing intervention.

Therapeutic Care Plan and Interventions

Following the client assessment, the nurse works with the client to establish goals for self-reflection. The plan should include self-reflection techniques that the client finds most appealing, and that both nurse and client agree will have the highest likelihood in helping to reach the goals.

BEFORE THE SESSION

- To be fully present with the client and with the intention to facilitate healing, begin with centering. This is done by engaging in deep breathing and systematic relaxation, letting go of other issues and concerns, and allowing yourself to be fully present in the moment with the client.
- Complete other physical treatments for the client and ensure the client's physical comfort prior to beginning a self-reflection intervention, so that the client may also be fully present in the moment and will not be distracted by physical sensations such as hunger or pain.
- Maintain privacy.
- Collect any special supplies required, such as paper, pencils, photograph albums, tape recorders, or music tapes, prior to initiating the intervention.

AT THE BEGINNING OF THE SESSION

- Begin the intervention by describing what is to be done and what the client may expect to achieve as a result of participating in the activity.

Exhibit 17-1 Nursing Interventions: Self-Reflection

Client Outcomes	Nursing Prescriptions	Evaluation
The client will demonstrate more effective coping skills as evident in weekly journal entries and clustering maps.	Guide the client in journal keeping and clustering to identify patterns of ineffective and effective coping skills.	The client demonstrates active problem solving and decreasing reliance on food and drugs.
The client will seek situations in which he or she interacts with others and will record feelings of belonging to a group through diary entries.	Guide the client to write daily about feelings and thoughts about the client and his or her relationships with others. Encourage the client to engage in lucid dreaming to imagine himself or herself interacting competently with others.	The client increases participation in social and family events and describes feelings of being more connected with others.
The client will reminisce about life through a life-review process and will verbalize a sense of meaning or purpose in life.	Facilitate six to eight sessions of reminiscence and life review in a support group setting. Encourage presentation of photographs and memorabilia.	The client states that, in addition to feeling sad about dying, he or she has come to realize that life has meaning and purpose and that he or she will be missed by family and friends.

- Begin with a relaxation exercise, including deep breathing and systematic muscle relaxation (see Chapter 21 for details).
- Encourage the client to quiet any inner chatter or dialogue that he or she may be experiencing, and to listen to his or her inner wisdom for guidance.
- If this is a second or subsequent session, review with the client events and situations that have transpired since the previous session before starting the relaxation exercise.

DURING THE SESSION

- Support the client through physical presence and encouragement.
- If the client requests solitude, respect this need and encourage the client to indicate when he or she is ready for further interaction.
- Encourage the client to ask questions, and clarify for the client the purpose and process involved in looking inward for wisdom and understanding.
- Monitor the environment to reduce stimuli in the form of noise, light, and odors that may distract the client from concentrating on the task at hand.
- Ensure that ample time and supplies are provided for the client to complete the strategies and obtain the maximum benefit from them.

AT THE END OF THE SESSION

- Before leaving the client, bring the client's focus back to the present time and place, reorienting the client as needed.
- Review what has been done and what goals have been met.

- Encourage the client to continue with homework, if needed, and provide for a mutually convenient time to review this homework.
- Assess the client's ability to continue reflective work on his or her own, and continue discussion if the client has difficulty in interpreting what has happened.

Specific Interventions: Self-Reflection

The purpose of self-reflection interventions is to help the client make sense of life events and circumstances that may be bewildering or discomforting.

KEEPING DIARIES OR JOURNALS

Keeping a diary or journal is a simple way to begin the process of self-reflection. Notes may be kept in a variety of forms, but a notebook or journal that keeps notes together in a single-bound format facilitates the use of these documents for review and for discerning patterns of response to life's events. Diaries may be structured or unstructured. Structuring diaries often facilitates the recording of information such as eating patterns, or patterns of pain and its management. Keeping a chart of symptoms, such as those associated with headache pain, may be useful in identifying interpersonal or environmental triggers for such symptoms. Unstructured diaries or journals provide the space to record thoughts and feelings about those situations that create anxiety or symptoms of illness. There is no correct or incorrect way to make entries in such a diary or journal; clients should be encouraged simply to allow themselves to follow their stream of consciousness and to play as they begin to write or draw in this format. The purpose is to release feelings, capture lessons learned in the past, apply those lessons to the present, and then connect the released feelings with thoughts, memories, beliefs, behaviors, and expectations about the future.

CREATING WORKS OF ART

Creating works of art, using methods such as drawing, sketching, painting, sculpting, weaving, sewing, or knitting, can be used to explore beliefs and shape outcomes.[1] To use one of these strategies for self-reflection, the client, with the nurse's help, identifies the purpose of the activity in terms of *process* rather than *product*. The purpose is to examine values and beliefs that may be hidden from conscious awareness, but that are influencing the client's experience of illness or disharmony. Images that emerge during the creative process are authentic and allow the individual to tap into wisdom that may lie beyond the client's usual ability to access.

WRITING LETTERS

Writing letters is a way to express a variety of feelings. While clients already may be writing letters to express positive feelings to others (e.g., by writing a thank-you note), they may be unaware of its usefulness as a strategy to express negative feelings such as anger and disappointment. The process of writing a letter is healing because it gives tangible expression to thoughts and feelings that are sometimes kept out of awareness. Letters that express negative emotions may be read aloud to another person, such as the nurse, who acts as a sounding board, or may be read for audio recording. After listening to the letter, the nurse may provide objective feedback, or the client may wish to listen to himself or herself on a tape recording. The letter then may be rewritten to clarify an expression of feelings.

BEGINNING AN INTUITION LOG

Intuition is a way of direct knowing that is not based on the usual linear method or rational analysis of sensory data.[2] Sudden flashes of insight that are unexpected are common experiences, but few people have learned to trust them as sources of truth or wisdom. Learning to trust such truths, however, contributes to healing and spiritual growth.[3] Some clients may benefit from carrying a personal intuition log with them. Each time they hear their inner voice, have a vague hunch, or experience a sudden "aha!" they can record it in the log book.[4]

USING METAPHORS

A metaphor is a word, phrase, or concept denoting one kind of idea that is used in place of another to suggest an analogy or similarity between the two.[5] This intervention helps clients deal with the questions "Who am I?" and "What is my life all about?" The purpose is to examine the meaning of a problem situation or of one's life in general by using a metaphor to describe some aspect of one's past, present, or future. Using an object to represent their life or an illness, clients are instructed to write or talk about themselves.

LEARNING FROM DREAMS

Dreams come from three different levels of consciousness: (1) the preconscious, which is the most readily accessible and contains material easily called into consciousness during the time one is awake; (2) the personal unconscious, which includes those memories that are generally hidden or repressed from waking consciousness, such as childhood traumas and fears; and (3) the collective unconscious, which includes the inherited aspects of mind that spawn the recurrent themes common in the mythology and legends of all cultures.

MIND MAPS AND CLUSTERING

Mind maps are a method for brainstorming by oneself. The purpose of this activity is to clarify one's thinking about a particular issue. As in group methods of brainstorming, four principles are involved: (1) judgment or evaluation of ideas should be suspended; (2) any idea or thought, no matter how illogical or absurd, is allowed; (3) the more ideas or thoughts generated, the better; and (4) all combinations or modifications of existing ideas are allowed.

USING THE MANDALA AND FOCUSING

The mandala, from the Sanskrit word meaning *circle*, is a ritualistic device used in Buddhism as a focus for meditation. Any circular geometric design can be used to focus the attention and quiet the inner dialogue. Focusing on such a harmonic symbol may serve as preparation for listening to the wisdom within.[6] Focusing may then be used to stimulate self-awareness and emotional healing by drawing attention to physical symptoms of illness or other bodily sensations.

SHARING STORIES

Each person's life is composed of stories. By telling stories about themselves, people can recreate who they are and who they will become. By sharing and hearing stories, people may develop a deeper understanding of themselves and the meaning of their lived experiences.[7]

REMINISCING AND EMBARKING ON A LIFE REVIEW

Life review is the process of consciously returning to past experiences, often including traumatic life events, that can be surveyed, resolved, and reintegrated into the self. The goal of this integration is the personal realization that life has been unique and has some kind of meaning.[8]

Evaluation

Periodically, the nurse and the client review the progress made toward achieving the goals or outcomes identified before beginning the self-reflection interventions. Many of the interventions described here take place over relatively long periods of time. Throughout the process, the nurse must monitor the client's progress and provide both presence and encouragement to continue the process of self-understanding and acceptance.

Nurse Healer Reflections

- What inner knowledge and awareness can be created by keeping a personal journal or dream diary?
- How can personal creativity and problem solving be enhanced by self-reflective techniques such as lucid dreaming or meditation?
- How can the life review process be used to ease the pain of death in clients?
- How can I learn to trust intuition in working with clients?

Notes

1. P.B. Allen, *Art Is a Way of Knowing* (Boston: Shambhala, 1995).
2. L. Rew, Intuition: Concept Analysis of a Group Phenomenon, *Advances in Nursing Science* 8, no. 2 (1986):21–28.
3. L. Rew, Intuition: Nursing Knowledge and the Spiritual Dimension of Persons, *Holistic Nursing Practice* 3, no. 3 (1989):56–68.
4. L.G. Kolkmeier, Self-Reflection: Consulting the Truth Within, in *Holistic Nursing: A Handbook for Practice*, 2nd ed., eds. B.M. Dossey et al. (Rockville, MD: Aspen Publishers, 1988).
5. The American Heritage Dictionary of the English Language, 4th ed. (Boston: Houghton Mifflin Company, 2000).
6. L. Rew, *Awareness in Healing* (Albany, NY: Delmar Publishers, 1996).
7. M.G. Nagai-Jacobson and M.A. Burkhardt, Viewing Persons as Stories: A Perspective for Holistic Care, *Alternative Therapies* 2, no. 4 (1996):54–58.
8. Nagai-Jacobson and Burkhardt, Viewing Persons as Stories.

Nutrition*

Nurse Healer Objective

- Explore each step of the holistic caring process when considering how nutrition can heal the bodymind.

Definitions

Antioxidants: substances that limit free radical formation and damage by stabilizing or deactivating free radicals before they attack cells.

Free Radicals: electrically charged molecules with an unpaired electron capable of attacking healthy cells in the body, causing them to lose their structure and function.

Glycemic Index: an index that classifies carbohydrate foods according to their glycemic response (effect on blood glucose levels), which varies with fiber content, starch structure, food processing, and presence of proteins and fats.

HDL: high-density lipoprotein form of cholesterol associated with reduced risk of atherosclerosis.

Homocysteine: an intermediate product of methionine metabolism and a marker for many clinical conditions, including cardiovascular disease.

* Condensed from: S. Luck, Nutrition, in *Holistic Nursing: A Handbook for Practice*, 4th ed., eds. B.M. Dossey, L. Keegan, C.E. Guzzetta (Sudbury, MA: Jones and Bartlett Publishers, 2005), 451–475.

LDL: low-density lipoprotein form of cholesterol strongly associated with increased risk of atherosclerosis.

Mineral: an inorganic trace element or compound that works in synergy with other compounds and is essential for human life.

Optimal Nutrition: adequate intake of nutrients for health promotion and disease prevention.

Phytochemicals: biologically active compounds found in foods.

Phytoestrogens: family of compounds found in plants that have some estrogenic and/or antiestrogenic activity in humans.

Probiotic: formulation containing beneficial living microorganisms that maintain health as part of the internal ecology of the digestive tract.

Vitamin: an organic substance necessary for normal growth, metabolism, and development of the body; acts as a catalyst and coenzyme, assisting in many chemical reactions while nourishing the body.

Xenoestrogens: synthetic, hormone-mimicking compounds found in certain pesticides, drugs, and plastics.

Healthy Choices in Nutrition

High-Fiber Diet

- whole grains: oatmeal, brown rice, millet, whole wheat, enriched pasta
- beans: lentils, tofu, split peas, garbanzo beans, black beans, tempeh
- vegetables: green, yellow, orange—steamed, raw, or stir-fried
- nuts and seeds: sunflower seeds, Brazil nuts, almonds, sesame seeds, pumpkin seeds, nut butters
- fruits: local and in season, such as papaya, melon, mango, grapefruit, berries

Note: Grains + beans = complete protein.

Low-Fat Diet

- Limit meats.
- Eliminate sandwich meats (ham, salami, bacon, sausage).
- Increase fish, chicken, turkey.
- Use cold-pressed, unprocessed oils—olive, canola, sesame.
- Use butter instead of margarine.
- Use low-fat dairy products.
- Bake, broil, steam, or poach food.

Foods To Avoid

- sugars—cookies, soda, candy, jelly, syrup
- processed foods—additives, preservatives, artificial colorings and flavorings
- canned foods—fresh is best, frozen is next best
- refined hydrogenated oils (Crisco, palm oil, cottonseed oil)
- fast foods and junk foods

Other Important Health Factors

- Drink four to six glasses of liquid daily—spring or filtered water, herbal teas.
- Cook and prepare food in cast-iron or stainless steel cookware (avoid aluminum).
- Chew foods slowly and thoroughly.
- Eat smaller, simpler meals.
- Include fiber with each meal.
- Exercise daily—walk, bicycle, jog, dance, swim, stretch.
- Reduce stress through yoga, meditation, deep breathing, relaxation practice, visualization.
- Avoid alcohol, caffeine, smoking, recreational drugs, over-the-counter drugs.
- Get sufficient rest and sleep.

Holistic Caring Process

Assessment

In preparing to use nutrition interventions, the nurse assesses the following parameters:

- the client's relationship to nutrition and diet: bio-chemical, genetic, cultural, social, emotional, religious, economic, environmental, and physiologic components
- the client's eating habits, food preferences, and nutritional needs
- the client's motivation and ability to make the necessary dietary and lifestyle changes
- the client's understanding that changing food and eating patterns is part of a wellness process

Patterns/Challenges/Needs

The following are the patterns/challenges/needs compatible with nutrition interventions that are related to the 13 domains of Taxonomy II (see Chapter 14):

- Altered nutrition
- Altered circulation
- Altered oxygenation
- Altered coping
- Altered physical mobility
- Sleep pattern disturbances
- Altered patterns of daily living
- Disturbance in body image
- Disturbance in self-esteem
- Potential hopelessness
- Potential powerlessness
- Knowledge deficit
- Pain

- Anxiety
- Grieving
- Depression
- Fear

Outcomes

Exhibit 18–1 guides the nurse in client outcomes, nursing pre-scriptions, and evaluation for the use of nutrition as a nursing intervention.

Therapeutic Care Plan and Interventions

BEFORE THE SESSION

- Create an environment in which the client feels com-fortable discussing physical and nutritional needs.
- Prepare assessment tools and educational materials.
- Focus on the client's nutritional and physical needs.
- Use relaxation techniques to assist the client before the session begins.

AT THE BEGINNING OF THE SESSION

- Take and record the necessary physical assessment data (e.g., weight, skin fold and thickness measurements).
- Guide the client to disclose past habit patterns that af-fect eating behavior.
- Have the client document food intake and association between food and feelings of well-being or distress.
- Assist the client in creating a sample menu.
- Encourage the client to participate in setting nutri-tional goals and action plans.
- Present specific nutritional guidelines for the client to follow.
- Direct the client to keep a food journal to present at follow-up session.

Exhibit 18-1 Nursing Interventions: Nutrition

Client Outcomes	Nursing Prescriptions	Evaluation
The client will be motivated to improve nutrition.	Assist the client in a personal self-assessment.	The client completed a self-assessment form.
	Encourage the client to participate with the nurse to develop goals and action plans.	The client participated with the nurse to develop a personalized program.
	Prepare the client to follow through with the nurse on evaluation and formulation of new goals.	The client met with the nurse for program evaluation.
The client will demonstrate knowledge of healthful nutrition.	Motivate the client to contribute to discussions about his or her program.	The client participated in the session discussion.
	Encourage the client to learn more about healthful behaviors as he or she works with the nurse.	The client demonstrated new knowledge.

DURING THE SESSION

- Have the nurse serve as a guide.
- Emphasize the connection between nutrition and whole-person health.
- With the nurse's guidance, have the client develop strategies for changing nutrition habits, nutrient intake, and eating patterns.
- Have the nurse assist the client in optimizing diet and nutrition by:
  — Creating an image for food as a healing medicine
  — Reframing the nutrition process into a positive action
  — Reframing nutrition and food as an empowerment tool
  — Illustrating how external nutrition changes promote internal healing responses
  — Reinforcing the client's positive changes in nutrition as part of the healing process
  — Ending sessions with images of desired state of well-being.

AT THE END OF THE SESSION

- Have the client identify the options presented that best fit with his or her own lifestyle.
- Work together with the client to write down goals and target dates.
- Give the client specific affirmations to use to support these goals.
- Give the client handout material to reinforce the teaching.
- Use the client outcomes that were established before the session (see Exhibit 18–1) and the client's subjective experiences (see Exhibit 18–2) to evaluate the session.
- Schedule a follow-up session.

Exhibit 18–2 Evaluation of the Client's Subjective Experience with Nutrition

1. Is this the first time you have considered the effects of healing nutrition from a holistic perspective?
2. Have you discovered ways you can eat for increased vitality and vibrant living?
3. Do you think there are any links between your food intake and the potential for development of a chronic disease in your life?
4. Is your life filled with healing foods? Do you want it to be?
5. What support systems would help you develop and adhere to a lifestyle that includes healing foods?
6. Can you think of anything else that would help you to maintain a routine that includes healing nutrition?
7. What is your next step (or your plan) to integrate these experiences on a daily basis?

Specific Interventions: Ensuring Optimal Nutrition

To optimize nutrient intake, the nurse may advise the client to

- adhere to recommended healthy diet
- practice relaxation techniques
- increase exercise following evaluation by a trained professional

The nurse can share information and research data on health benefits of antioxidants and other nutrients known to assist in the health and healing process.

A daily menu plan can be created to fit the client's particular needs. The following should be considered:

- daily activity status
- current health status

- any physical limitations
- economic considerations
- social and cultural influences
- emotion state of being
- individual differences, including food preferences and religious dietary customs

To motivate and assist the client, the nurse can

- encourage the client to write a food journal daily
- demonstrate the daily practice of asking the body what it needs to be healthy
- create daily menus using healthy choices that are mutually agreed upon
- teach the client to self-assess health changes that occur with dietary interventions
- encourage the client who is currently using nutritional supplementation to organize a routine to optimize compliance and benefits

Open-ended questions, images, journal writing, drawing, and other creative strategies to integrate nutrition into the client's daily life can be used to close the session.

Evaluation

Nurses should chart all information they impart to the client, as well as an evaluation of the session. When the nurse works in an inpatient facility, other staff need to be appraised of the program and its progress. Nurses who work in wellness centers, in centers using integrated models, and in private practice should also keep records for each client and should state nursing diagnosis, type of counseling employed, and the effectiveness of each session.

The nurse is in a prime position to model the effects of healthy nutrition and lifestyle by integrating these elements into daily life and practicing self-care.

Nurse Healer Reflections

- What sensations accompany physical well-being because of my improved nutrition?
- What comprises healthy eating for both myself and my clients?
- How can I model healthy nutrition practices?

Exercise and Movement*

Nurse Healer Objective

- Explore each step of the holistic caring process when considering exercise and movement.

Definitions

Aerobic Exercise: sustained muscle activity within the target heart range that challenges the cardiovascular system to meet the muscles' needs for oxygen.

Anaerobic Exercise: exercise that is fueled by the energy within the muscles used.

Endurance: the period of time the body can sustain exercise or movement.

Fitness: the ability to carry out daily tasks with vigor and alertness, without undue fatigue, and with ample reserve to enjoy leisure pursuits; the ability to respond to physical and emotional stress without an excessive increase in heart rate and blood pressure.

Flexibility: the ability to use a joint throughout its full range of motion and to maintain some degree of elasticity of major muscle groups.

Kinetic Energy: energy associated with motion, energizing, or dynamic energy.

Maximal Heart Rate: the rate of the heart when the body is engaged in intense physical activity.

---

* Condensed from: B.H. Cricket Rose and L. Keegan, Exercise and Movement, in *Holistic Nursing: A Handbook for Practice*, 4th ed., eds. B.M. Dossey, L. Keegan, C.E. Guzzetta (Sudbury, MA: Jones and Bartlett Publishers, 2005), 479–493.

Movement: changes in the spatial configuration of the body and its parts, such as in breathing, eating, speaking, gesturing, and exercising; motion away from mental, physical, emotional, or spiritual stasis.

Nonaerobic Exercise: sustained physical activity above the normal resting state that uses one or more major muscle groups, but that is not intense enough to cause an increased muscle oxygen uptake.

Posture: pose, or placement of parts of the body in spatial relationships.

Resistance Training: the use of weights or opposing forces to exercise (strengthen) muscle groups.

Resting Heart Rate: the rate of the heart when the body is in deep rest.

Strength: the power of muscle groups.

Target Heart Rate: the safe rate for the heart during exercise.

Training: repetitive bouts of exercise over a period of time with the intention of developing fitness.

Holistic Caring Process

Assessment

In preparing to use exercise and movement interventions, the nurse assesses the following parameters:

- the client's financial and religious restrictions, as well as habit patterns formed during childhood, and cultural approaches to exercise and movement
- the client's nonverbal movement patterns and known movement limitations
- the client's motivation, desire, and ability to make the necessary lifestyle changes in the areas of exercise and movement

Patterns/Challenges/Needs

The following are the patterns/challenges/needs compatible with the interventions for exercise and movement that are related to the 13 domains of Taxonomy II (see Chapter 14):

- Altered nutrition
- Altered circulation
- Altered oxygenation
- Altered coping
- Altered physical mobility
- Sleep pattern disturbance
- Altered activities of daily living
- Disturbance in body image
- Disturbance in self-esteem
- Potential hopelessness
- Potential powerlessness
- Knowledge deficit
- Pain
- Anxiety
- Grieving

Outcomes

Exhibit 19–1 guides the nurse in client outcomes, nursing prescriptions, and evaluation for the use of exercise and movement as nursing interventions.

Therapeutic Care Plan and Interventions

BEFORE THE SESSION

- Create an environment in which the client feels comfortable discussing the needs of his or her physical body from a physical movement perspective.
- Clear your mind of other client or personal encounters in order to be fully present when meeting with the client.

Exhibit 19-1 Nursing Interventions: Exercise and Movement

Client Outcomes	Nursing Prescriptions	Evaluation
The client will be motivated to improve exercise and movement practice.	Assist the client in a personal self-assessment.	The client completed a self-assessment form.
	Encourage the client to participate with the nurse to develop goals and action plans.	The client participated with the nurse to develop a personalized program of exercise and movement.
	Prepare the client to follow through with the nurse on evaluation and formulation of new goals.	The client met with the nurse to evaluate program results.
The client will demonstrate knowledge of healthful exercise and movement programs and resources.	Motivate the client to contribute to discussions about his or her program.	The client participated in the session discussions.
	Encourage the client to learn more about healthful behaviors as he or she works with the nurse.	The client demonstrated content knowledge and resource acquisition for using new behaviors in exercise and movement programs.

- Gather input data forms and teaching charts.
- Prepare all necessary assessment equipment.
- Prepare handouts or between-session worksheets to give to the client during the session.

AT THE BEGINNING OF THE SESSION

- Take and record the necessary physical assessment data (e.g., height, weight, skin-fold thickness measurements, body contour measurements, blood pressure, data on range of motion and mobility limitations).
- Guide the client as he or she discloses past habit patterns that affect exercise behavior.

DURING THE SESSION

- Review with the client current weekly exercise patterns.
- Be alert to psychologic clues that may relate to exercise behavior or extremes (exhaustion versus training versus sedentariness).
- Following data collection, work with the client to develop an individualized exercise and movement program.
- Make certain that teaching is at the client's intellectual and emotional level.

AT THE END OF THE SESSION

- Have the client identify the options presented that best fit his or her lifestyle.
- Work with the client to write down goals and target dates.
- Give the client specific affirmations to use to support these goals.
- Give the client handout material to reinforce the teaching.
- Use the client outcomes that were established before the session (see Exhibit 19–1) and the client's subjective experiences (see Exhibit 19–2) to evaluate the session.
- Schedule a follow-up session.

Exhibit 19-2 Evaluation of the Client's Subjective Experience with Exercise and Movement Interventions

1. Is this the first time you have experimented with your exercise routine?
2. Have you experienced any sense of release during the changed physical activity?
3. Has your vitality increased since beginning regular exercise?
4. Does exercise give you a sense of reduced stress in your life?
5. Do you find time during your normal day to integrate special movement techniques?
6. If not, would you like to learn more ways to improve your movement periods at work?
7. What support systems have you discovered that assist you with maintaining and developing your exercise regimen?
8. Is there some other support that you need to assist you in adhering to your new exercise regimen?
9. What is your next step for integrating exercise and therapeutic movement into your daily life?
10. Do you need help in obtaining more resources for this final step?

Specific Interventions: Exercise and Movement

EXERCISE (BASIC)

The primary purpose of exercise is to produce fitness. The basic components of fitness are:

1. Flexibility—the ability to use a joint throughout its full range of motion and to maintain some degree of elasticity of major muscle groups. It is important because
   • it provides increased resistance to muscle and joint injury
   • it helps prevent mild muscle soreness if flexibility exercises are done before and after vigorous activity

2. Muscle strength—the contracting power of a muscle. It is important because
   - daily activities become less strenuous as muscles become stronger
   - strong abdominal and lower back muscles help prevent lower back problems
   - appearance improves as muscles become firmer
3. Cardiorespiratory endurance—the ability of the circulatory and respiratory systems to maintain blood and oxygen delivery to the exercising muscles. It is important because
   - it increases resistance to cardiovascular diseases
   - it improves the ability to maintain activity levels
   - it allows for a high energy return for daily activities
4. Postural stability—the body's ability to balance and stay balanced during dynamic action. This ability declines naturally with age; exercise continuation assists with preventing falls through integration of neuromuscular and sensory responses.

To reduce risks associated with exercise, you must know not only how often and how long to exercise but also how vigorously to exercise. Although the target pulse range allows for a heart rate within 60 to 80 percent of maximal capacity, the American Heart Association guidelines state that regular exercise of a moderate level, or from 50 to 75 percent of maximal capacity, appears to be sufficient. Maintaining the target pulse rate during physical exercise for 15 to 30 minutes three to five times per week reduces the risk of overexertion, enhances enjoyment, and results in cardiovascular fitness.

MOVEMENT (BASIC)

There are four components of creative movement: centering, warm-up, exploration of surrounding space, and stretching.

1. Centering is the inward focusing on one's own physical reality. The duration of this process varies, but it usually lasts 3 to 10 minutes.
2. The stretching, breathing warm-up exercises follow the centering exercise and are designed to "wake up" the muscles while maintaining the harmonious integration of psyche and soma that was begun through centering.
3. Exploration of surrounding space occurs as movement proceeds and there is an awakened sense of self-awareness. With this discovery of new physical capacities comes increased kinetic and spatial awareness. During this time, there may be swinging, swaying, and laughter.
4. Stretching concludes a dance movement, allowing for relaxation as it brings one to a resting state. At the conclusion, one should savor the feeling of energetic relaxation.

Evaluation

Attention to exercise and movement can lead to a general improvement of health and decrease the risk factors of major diseases. The nurse is in a prime position to model the effects of healthy exercise and movement behaviors.

Nurse Healer Reflections

- How would I describe the place of movement and exercise in my life today?
- What mental or spiritual sensations accompany my physical sensations because of my improved exercise and movement status?
- How should I feel when I am physically fit?
- What exercise and movement changes can I incorporate in my daily life to improve my fitness?
- How can I learn, practice, and model healthy exercise and movement?

CHAPTER 20

Humor, Laughter, and Play*

Nurse Healer Objective

- Explore each step of the holistic caring process when considering humor, laughter, and play.

Definitions

Humor: a quality of perception and attitude toward life that enables an individual to experience joy even when facing adversity; a perception of the absurdity or incongruity of a situation.

Laughter: a physical behavior that occurs in response to something that is perceived as humorous, amusing, or surprising. This behavior engages most of the muscle groups and organ systems within the body. Laughter is often preceded by physical, emotional, or cognitive tension.

Play: a spontaneous or recreational activity that is performed for sheer enjoyment rather than to reach a goal or produce a product. Playfulness is a mood or attitude that infuses the individual with a sense of joy and positive emotions.

---

* Condensed from: P. Wooten, Humor, Laughter, and Play, in *Holistic Nursing: A Handbook for Practice*, 4th ed., eds. B.M. Dossey, L. Keegan, C.E. Guzzetta (Sudbury, MA: Jones and Bartlett Publishers, 2005), 497–520.

Holistic Caring Process

Assessment

In preparing to use humor, laughter, and play interventions, the nurse assesses the following parameters:

- the client's ability and willingness to smile and laugh
- the client's attitude toward using laughter and play in the current situation
- the client's history of using humor, laughter, and play in other circumstances
- the client's visual, auditory, cognitive, and physical limitations
- the client's preferred style of humor
- the client's favorite comedy artists—performers, writers, cartoonists, and so on
- the client's feelings about previous experiences with humor and play
- the client's preferred playful activities

Patterns/Challenges/Needs

The following are the patterns/challenges/needs compatible with the interventions for humor, laughter, and play that are related to the 13 domains of Taxonomy II (see Chapter 14):

- Altered parenting, actual or potential
- Social isolation
- Ineffective individual and family coping
- Activity intolerance, actual or potential
- Deficit in diversional activity
- Impaired physical mobility
- Powerlessness
- Disturbance in self-concept: altered self-esteem, role performance, personal identity
- Altered sensation/perception: visual, auditory, kinesthetic, gustatory, tactile, olfactory

- Altered thought processes
- Anxiety
- Pain
- Fear
- Potential for violence: self-directed or directed at others

Outcomes

Exhibit 20–1 guides the nurse in outcomes, nursing prescriptions, and evaluation for the use of humor, laughter, and play as a nursing intervention.

Therapeutic Care Plan and Interventions

BEFORE THE SESSION

- Assess your own ease and comfort with using humor and play as a therapeutic intervention.
- Practice smiling in front of a mirror. First scowl, then smile. Feel the difference.
- Evaluate your ability to respond to humor or engage in playful activity for your own personal pleasure.
- Increase awareness of your own preferred humor style, artist, writer, performer.
- Allow yourself to laugh with abandon at things you find funny.
- Become familiar with the content and variety of humorous items and playful activities that are available for you to use.
- Ensure that all supplies and equipment are in working condition.
- Improve your ability to tell a good joke. Remember these tips: Keep it short—less than 2 minutes. Be sure you can remember the whole joke before you start. Let your body, face, and voice become animated as you tell the joke. Pause occasionally as you deliver the material; create a brief and concise setup for the punch line;

Exhibit 20-1 Nursing Interventions: Play and Laughter

Client Outcomes	Nursing Prescriptions	Evaluation
The client will smile and/or laugh in response to humorous stimuli.	Introduce the client to the concept that humor, laughter, and play benefit health.	The client requested some humor resources from family or friends.
	Guide the client in identifying his or her own preferred humor style.	The client laughed in response to a selected humorous intervention.
	Help the client to clarify any blocks to using humor, laughter, or play.	The client laughed at a joke, story, or cartoon provided by the nurse.
		The client shared a joke or story with the nurse or family.
		The client sees some absurdity in a personal incident and shares with staff or family.
The client will engage in playful activities.	Guide client to select a playful activity that matches his or her preference and ability.	The client was observed amusing self with toy.
		The client plays game with family during visiting hours.
		The client wears amusing item to greet staff or family.
The client will experience decrease in subjective severity of target symptom as a result of humor or playful intervention.	Guide client in grading the severity of a symptom on a scale of 1 to 10 before and after intervention.	Patient rated pain at 6 before humor intervention and graded pain at 3 after intervention.

pause before delivering the punch line; speak the punch line clearly and with punch!
- Review the client's chart or consult with others to assess changes in the client's situation since you last met.
- Sense your own needs and stress level. Give yourself permission to be silly and playful.

AT THE BEGINNING OF THE SESSION
- Assess the client's status according to the assessment parameters.
- Record vital signs and ask the client to assess pain, anxiety, tension, or other target symptoms on a numerical scale (1 = comfortable, 10 = extremely uncomfortable).
- Describe to the client the benefits that humor, laughter, and play have on the body (physiologic), mind (psychologic), and spirit (emotional and energy level).
- Provide the client with appropriate materials to match his or her preference and some instructions for use.

DURING THE SESSION
- Use all interventions with sensitivity to the client's needs, response, and difficulties.
- Provide support for the client through your physical presence, encouragement, or time alone if the client wants to read or watch a videotape.
- Remember that humor is contagious and social. Interventions may be most effective if used within a group (e.g., family and friends) rather than individually.
- Remember that humor and play are spontaneous and therefore are most successful when not precisely planned.
- Continue to evaluate the mood and response of the client and adapt the humor and play intervention to meet the client's perceived needs.

AT THE END OF THE SESSION

- Record vital signs and ask the client to reevaluate the pain, tension, or target symptom on a scale of 1 to 10.
- Discuss the intervention with the client and obtain feedback for future sessions.
- Answer any questions the client may have.
- Encourage the client to continue using the intervention at home and to explore other possible variations.
- Use client outcomes (Exhibit 20–1) and the client's subjective experiences (Exhibit 20–2) to evaluate the session.
- Schedule a follow-up session.

Specific Interventions: Humor, Laughter, and Play

Humor interventions can be packaged in many different ways—as humor rooms, comedy carts, humor baskets, laughter libraries, or caring clown programs. The individual caregiver

---

Exhibit 20-2 Evaluation of the Client's Subjective Experience with Humor, Laughter, and Play

1. Was this a new experience for you? Can you describe it?
2. Can you describe any physical or emotional shift that occurred during the exercise?
3. Were there any distractions or uncomfortable moments during the exercise?
4. How long has it been since you had this kind of experience?
5. How was this exercise different for you from the last time you took part in a similar one?
6. Would you like to try this again?
7. How could the experience be made more meaningful for you?
8. What are your plans to integrate this exercise into your daily life?

can adapt these programs to meet the specific needs of clients. Several suggestions for starting a humor program follow:

- Create a scrapbook of cartoons. Place the cartoons in a photo album with peel-back pages to protect them and keep them clean. Consider the audience that will read this scrapbook. Try to find humor about situations or problems your clients will be facing. Be careful not to add any potentially offensive or shocking items to the scrapbook. Include a variety of cartoon artists.
- Develop a file of funny jokes, stories, cards, bumper stickers, poems, and songs.
- Collect or borrow funny books, DVDs, videos, and audio cassettes of comedy routines. These can be found in libraries, humor sections of bookstores, mail-order catalogs, or at humor conferences.
- Keep a file of local clowns, magicians, storytellers, and puppeteers. Invite them to entertain at your facility, at the patient's home, or at a group function.
- Collect toys, interactive games, noisemakers, and costume items. Keep them available for play. Small wind-up toys can be enjoyable. The author has a pair of little shoes that walk around when wound up and a large nose that does the same—it is called the "runny nose." If you will be sharing such toys with a client, keep in mind safety and infection precautions.
- Create a humor journal or log to record funny encounters or humorous discoveries. On days when you really need a laugh but cannot seem to find anything funny, you will have a collection of amusing stories at your fingertips.
- Establish a bulletin board in your facility or on your refrigerator at home. Post cartoons, bumper stickers, and funny signs. If the display is public, you must consider the sensitivities of the audience and be careful to ex-

clude potentially offensive (e.g., ageist, sexist, ethnic) material.

- Subscribe to a humorous newsletter or journal to collect new ideas and inspiration.

- Educate yourself about therapeutic humor. Attend conferences, workshops, and conventions. New techniques are developed daily. New research is published, and better resources become available on a regular basis. Stay up-to-date in this rapidly growing field.

Evaluation

With the client, the nurse determines whether the client outcomes for humor, laughter, and play (see Exhibit 20–1) were successfully achieved. To evaluate the session further, the nurse may again explore the subjective effects of the experience with the client using the evaluation questions in Exhibit 20–2.

Nurse Healer Reflections

- What is my inner sense of joy when I hear myself or another laugh?

- Do I nurture my ability, and the ability of my patients, to be playful?

- Can I laugh and play with a sense of freedom and without guilt, even when my work is not yet finished?

- Can I experience playful activities without competing, or feeling that I must accomplish a particular goal?

CHAPTER 21

Relaxation: The First Step to Restore, Renew, and Self-Heal*

Nurse Healer Objective

- Explore each step of the holistic caring process when using relaxation with various clients to facilitate the healing process.

Definitions

Autogenic Training: self-directed therapy that focuses on repetition of phrases about desired states of the body (e.g., heaviness and warmth).

Mantra: a word, short phrase, or prayer that is repeated either silently or aloud as a focus of concentration during the practice of meditation.

Meditation: originally based in spiritual traditions, the practice of focusing and concentrating one's attention and awareness while maintaining a passive attitude; evolves with discipline and practice and is known for providing health benefits as well as being a road to spiritual transformation.

* Condensed from: J. Anselmo, Relaxation: The First Step to Restore, Renew, and Self-Heal, in *Holistic Nursing: A Handbook for Practice*, 4th ed., eds. B.M. Dossey, L. Keegan, C.E. Guzzetta (Sudbury, MA: Jones and Bartlett Publishers, 2005), 523–564.

Note: The author would like to acknowledge previous contributions of Leslie Gooding Kolkmeier as the originator of this chapter in its first edition, as well as being co-author in previous editions.

Pain (Medical Definition): localized sensation of hurt, or an unpleasant sensory and emotional experience associated with actual or potential tissue damage, or described in terms of such damage.

Pain (Nursing Definition): a subjective experience including both verbal and nonverbal behavior.[1]

Progressive Muscle Relaxation: the process of alternately tensing and relaxing muscle groups to become aware of subtle degrees of tension and relaxation; originally developed by Edmund Jacobson.

Relaxation: a psychophysiologic experience characterized by parasympathetic dominance involving multiple visceral and somatic systems; the absence of physical, mental, and emotional tension; the opposite of Canon's "fight or flight" response and Selye's general adaptation syndrome.[2]

Relaxation Response: an alert, hypokinetic process of decreased sympathetic nervous system arousal that may be achieved in a number of ways, including through breathing exercises, relaxation and imagery exercises, biofeedback, and prayer. A degree of discipline is required to evoke this response, which increases mental and physical well-being.

Self-Hypnosis: an approach for voluntarily fostering a consciousness process for the purpose of influencing one's thoughts, perceptions, behaviors, or sensations.

Stress (Psychophysiologic Definition): the felt experience of overactivity of the sympathetic nervous system.

Holistic Caring Process

Assessment

In preparing to use relaxation interventions, the nurse assesses the following parameters and lived experiences:

- the client's perception of personal tension levels and need to relax.

- the client's readiness and motivation to learn relaxation strategies.
- the client's past experience with the process of relaxation.
- the client's personal definition and lived experience of what it means to be relaxed.
- the client's ability to remain comfortably in one position for 15 to 30 minutes.
- the client's hearing acuity.
- the client's religious beliefs.
- the client's level of pain or discomfort.
- the client's medication intake, particularly of medications that may alter response to relaxation or that may need to be titrated as relaxation progresses.

Patterns/Challenges/Needs

The following are the patterns/challenges/needs compatible with relaxation interventions that are related to the 13 domains of Taxonomy II (see Chapter 14):

- Social isolation
- Altered coping; ineffective individual and family
- Activity intolerance, actual or potential
- Deficit in diversional activity
- Powerlessness
- Altered self-concept; disturbance in self-esteem, role performance, personal identity
- Altered sensation/perception: visual, auditory, kinesthetic, gustatory, tactile, olfactory
- Altered thought processes
- Anxiety
- Altered comfort: pain
- Fear
- Potential for violence: self-directed or directed at others

Outcomes

Exhibit 21–1 guides the nurse in client outcomes, nursing prescriptions, and evaluations for the use of relaxation as a nursing intervention.

Therapeutic Care Plan and Interventions

BEFORE THE SESSION

- Review with the client his or her lived experience concerning pain, anxiety, and activity levels.

PREPARATION OF THE ENVIRONMENT (IDEAL)

- Arrange medical and nursing care to allow for 15 to 45 minutes of uninterrupted time.
- Keep the room warm and ventilated, not cold.
- Shut the door.
- Unplug the telephone.
- Reduce lighting to a low level.
- Use natural or incandescent lighting if possible.

CLIENT COMFORT MEASURES

- Have the client empty his or her bladder.
- Help the client find a comfortable sitting or reclining position.
- Ensure the client's comfort by providing a blanket; have small, soft pillows available for positioning.

TIMING OF THE SESSION (IDEAL)

- Hold the training session before meals or more than 2 hours after the last meal.

SUPPORT TOOLS

- Have available music tapes/CDs.

Exhibit 21-1 Nursing Interventions: Relaxation

Client Outcomes	Nursing Prescriptions	Evaluation
The client will demonstrate decreased anxiety, tension, and other manifestations of the stress response as a result of the relaxation intervention.	Guide the client in the relaxation exercise. Evaluate for decrease in anxiety, tension, and other manifestations of the stress response as evidenced by normal heart rate within normal limits, decreased respiratory rates, return of blood pressure toward normal, resolution of anxious facial expressions and mannerisms, decrease in repetitious talking or behavior, and ability to sleep.	The client exhibited decreased anxiety, tension, and other manifestations of the stress response as evidenced by normal vital signs; a slow, deep breathing pattern; and decreased anxious behaviors.
The client will demonstrate a stabilization or decrease in pain as a result of the relaxation intervention.	Evaluate for decrease in pain as evidenced by reduction or elimination of pain control medication and increased activities or mobility.	The client's intake of pain medication stabilized and then decreased with relaxation skills practice. The client began to participate in activities previously limited by pain.
The client will link breathing awareness to a commonly occurring cue and use this combination to reduce tension.	Teach awareness of breathing patterns and habitual linking of relaxing breathing to a cue in the environment.	The client used turning in bed as a cue to take a slow, deep breath and relax jaw muscles.

- Tell the client that you may ask simple yes or no questions that they may answer by raising a preestablished 'yes' finger or 'no' finger or nodding the head.

AT THE BEGINNING OF THE SESSION

- Review briefly the potential benefits of relaxation intervention and enlist the client's cooperation (Exhibit 21–2). Explore the client's lived experience of relaxation and stress (Exhibit 21–3).
- Explain to the client that relaxation may be easier if practiced with the eyes closed.
- Explain that one purpose of breathing and relaxation exercises is to experience inward relaxation.
- Emphasize that you are merely a guide, and that any therapeutic results obtained from the session are due to the client's involvement, interest, and practice.
- Let go of outcomes. Encourage the client to practice for comfort and awareness, noting shifts in breathing, anxiety, and sensations.
- Arrive at mutually agreeable goals for the session.
- Have the client quantify the level of the parameter to be changed; for example, "My pain or anxiety level right now is 7 on a scale of 0 (none) to 10 (extreme pain)." Record the level before and after the session.
- Record baseline vital signs. If biofeedback equipment is used, record baseline readings.
- Assure the client that sensations of heaviness, warmth, floating, or lightness are naturally occurring indications of deep relaxation.
- Begin soft background music.
- Guide the client through a basic breathing relaxation exercise.
- Start the session with short breathing or relaxation exercises (5 minutes).

Exhibit 21-2 Clinical Benefits of Relaxation

Relaxation training has the following clinical benefits:

- decreasing the anxiety accompanying painful situations, such as debridement or dressing changes
- easing the muscle tension pain of skeletal muscle contractions
- decreasing fatigue by interrupting the fight or flight response
- providing a period of rest as beneficial as a nap
- helping the client fall asleep quickly
- increasing the effect of pain medications
- helping the client dissociate from pain

DURING THE SESSION

- Phrase all therapeutic suggestions and self-statements in a positive form. For example, say "I am aware of comfort moving down my arm and into my hand," rather than, "I am not in pain."
- Speak in a relaxed manner.
- Pace your instructions according to the following visual cues from the client:
  — change in breathing pattern: slower, deeper breaths progressing to slow, somewhat shallower breathing as relaxation deepens
  — more audible breathing
  — fluttering of eyelids
  — blanching of the skin around the nose and mouth
  — easing of jaw tightness
  — if client is supine, pointing of toes outward rather than straight up
- Modify your instructions and strategies to fit the situation.

Exhibit 21-3   Important Factors in Relaxation Practice

- **Passive volition:** Letting go, being without doing or striving, allowing, being with the process as it unfolds rather than making it happen; planting a seed in the mind of wanting to relax and then letting go and watching the process.

- **Attention to the here and now:** Being oriented toward the present, not caught up in what happened or what might happen.

- **Altered perception of time:** Experiencing time as expanded or contracted. Relaxation practice can change the perception of time so that a very short practice session feels like a long time or a long practice session is experienced as a few moments.

- **Enjoyment of practice:** Committing to practice and, even more importantly, enjoying practice. Most traditional healers and teachers of the restorative arts ask their students if they are enjoying their practice. Finding a practice that helps one weather the storms of life and enhances one's inner connection is a joy.

- Intersperse your instructions with therapeutic suggestions of encouragement that the client can use after the session as cues to recapture aspects of the relaxation experience.
- Be alert for signs of emotional discomfort or letting go, such as tears or a change in breathing to deeper, faster breaths.

AT THE END OF THE SESSION

- Bring the client gradually into a wakeful state by suggesting that he or she take deep, energizing breaths, begin to move hands and feet, and stretch; orient the client to the room, talking with the client about the comfort he or she created.

- Have the client reevaluate, on the scale of 0 to 10 used earlier, the level of comfort or severity of the parameter previously selected to be changed. Record the level.
- Allow time for discussion of the experience.

Evaluation

With the client, the nurse determines whether the client outcomes for relaxation interventions (see Exhibit 21–1) were successfully achieved. To evaluate the session further, the nurse may again explore the subjective effects of the experience with the client (Exhibit 21–4).

Nurse Healer Reflections

- How do I model relaxation to my family, friends, colleagues, and clients?
- What cues about my inner experience of tension or relaxation do I receive from my breathing pattern?

Exhibit 21–4   Evaluation of the Client's Subjective Experience of Relaxation

1. Was this a new experience for you? Can you describe it?
2. Did you have any physical or emotional responses to the relaxation exercises? If so, can you describe them?
3. Do you feel different after this experience? How?
4. How does your bodymind communicate with you when your stress level is at an uncomfortable point?
5. Would you like to do this again?
6. Were there any distractions to your relaxation?
7. What would make this a more pleasant experience for you?
8. How do you see yourself integrating relaxation skills into your daily life?

Notes

1. N. Meinhart and M. McCaffery, *Pain: A Nursing Approach to Assessment and Analysis* (East Norwalk, CT: Appleton-Century-Crofts, 1983), 377.

2. K. Phillips, Biofeedback as an Aid to Autogenic Training, in *Mind and Cancer Prognosis*, ed. B. Stoll (New York: John Wiley & Sons, 1979), 153.

CHAPTER 22

Imagery: Awakening the Inner Healer*

Nurse Healer Objective
- Explore each step of the holistic caring process when using imagery with various clients to facilitate the healing process.

Definitions

Clinical Imagery: the conscious use of the power of the imagination with the intention of activating physiological, psychological, or spiritual healing.

End-State Imagery: images that contain specified imagined hopes and goals (e.g., a healed wound).

Guided Imagery: a highly structured imagery technique.

Imagery Process: internal experiences of memories, dreams, fantasies, inner perceptions, and visions, sometimes involving one, several, or all of the senses, serving as the bridge for connecting body, mind, and spirit.

Visualization: the use of external images (e.g., religious painting, written word, nature photograph) to evoke internal imagery experiences that energize desired emotions, qualities, outcomes, or goals.

---

* Condensed from: B.G. Schaub, B.M. Dossey, Imagery: Awakening the Inner Healer, in *Holistic Nursing: A Handbook for Practice*, 4th ed., eds. B.M. Dossey, L. Keegan, C.E. Guzzetta (Sudbury, MA: Jones and Bartlett Publishers, 2005), 567–613.

Imagery

Imagery is an essential aspect of holistic nursing practice, as it brings the natural powers of the mind into the process of health and healing.[1,2,3] Distinct from thinking, imagery as a technique interacts with the image-making function of the brain, which in turn acts on the entire physiology. Imagery can be used on its own or in conjunction with therapeutic touch, meditation, biofeedback, reiki, reflexology, and other holistic practices. Imagery is an independent nursing intervention, a nurse-initiated action performed by nurses to bring about patient outcomes falling within the scope of nursing practice.

Holistic Caring Process

Assessment

In preparing to use imagery as a nursing intervention, the nurse assesses the following parameters:

- the client's potential for organic brain syndrome or psychosis in order to determine if general relaxation techniques should be used instead of imagery techniques.
- the client's anxiety/tension levels in order to determine which types of relaxation inductions will be most effective.
- the client's hopes in regard to the session and reason for seeking help.
- the client's understanding that it is not necessary to literally hear, see, feel, touch, or taste when working with imagery; that it is best to trust the inner experience in whatever form the information comes.

Patterns/Challenges/Needs

The following are the patterns/challenges/needs compatible with imagery interventions that are related to the 13 domains of Taxonomy II (see Chapter 14):

- Pain
- Anxiety
- Spiritual distress
- Altered effective coping
- Potential for growth
- Health-seeking behaviors

- Sleep pattern disturbance
- Potential hopelessness
- Potential powerlessness
- Fear
- Grief

Outcomes

Exhibit 22–1 guides the nurse in client outcomes, nursing prescriptions, and evaluations for the use of imagery as a nursing intervention.

Therapeutic Care Plan and Implementation

BEFORE THE SESSION

- Become calm and centered. Prepare to guide the client with relaxation induction (see Chapter 21) and imagery.
- Have the client sit, recline, or lie down, depending on client preference and clinical situation.
- Have a selection of music tapes available from which the client can choose (see Chapter 23).

AT THE BEGINNING OF THE SESSION

- Give the client a general definition of imagery: "Imagery is a natural way to connect body-mind-spirit by quieting the busy mind and body. This helps you tap into the power of the imagination."
- Assist the client in experiencing the imagery process and making friends with the experience of inner wisdom. This process is a key aspect of self-empowerment and creativity.

DURING THE SESSION

- Guide the client with specific emerging scripts or invite him or her to use personal images.
- Assess the state of relaxation throughout the session.

Exhibit 22-1   Nursing Interventions: Imagery

Client Outcomes	Nursing Prescriptions	Evaluation
The client will demonstrate skills in imagery.	Following an assessment, guide the client in an imagery exercise.	The client participated in imagery exercise by choice.
	Assess the client's levels of anxiety with this new process.	The client demonstrated no signs of anxiety with imagery process.
	After the imagery process experience, assess effectiveness through client dialogue.	The client stated that the imagery experience was helpful.
	Encourage the client to recognize daily self-talk and the images that lead to balance and inner peace.	The client reported using self-dialogue with imagery.
	Help the client to create images of desired health habits, feelings, desires for daily living.	The client reported creating images of desired health habits, feelings, and desires for daily living.
	Teach the client coping, power over daily events, ability to move toward healthy lifestyle.	The client reported increased coping with daily stressors.
	Teach the client to recognize images leading to self-defeating lifestyle habits.	The client reported recognition of negative images leading to self-defeating behavior; the client created positive images.

AT THE END OF THE SESSION

- Bring the client to an alert state gradually, allowing time for silence before discussion. Observe and take cues from the client as to the appropriate time to begin the discussion related to imagery session.
- Introduce the idea of "constant instant practice," using some frequent activity of daily life (e.g., telephone calls) as a reminder to practice imagery.
- Schedule a follow-up session.

Specific Interventions

FACILITATION AND INTERPRETATION OF THE IMAGERY PROCESS

In order to facilitate the imagery process, the nurse serves as a guide.[4] There is absolutely no way to predict what will surface in a client's imagination. Every experience is different, even when the same script is used. Nurses who are unfamiliar with imagery and guiding should learn a few basic relaxation and imagery scripts, and practice on themselves by making tapes of their own voice and following their own guiding. This will help build confidence with the intervention. It is helpful to learn a variety of scripts pertaining to common problems in clinical practice, such as preoperative anxiety, recovery from surgery, postoperative coughing, effective wound healing, fear, anxiety, pain, and relationship problems.

GUIDED IMAGERY SCRIPTS

The guidelines that follow will help the nurse in the effective implementation of imagery scripts as nursing interventions:[5]

- Start the session with an induction, a general relaxation—focusing on breath, shortened passive progressive relaxation, or body awareness, for example (also see Chapter 21).

- Reaffirm that there is no right or wrong way for the client to do imagery, that whatever occurs is useful information, and that the client has complete control over the process (e.g., deciding whether to go further or to stop).
- Personalize the imagery by using the client's name or other specific references several times during the process.

General Imagery

Scripts:
- *Let your imagination choose a place that is safe and comfortable . . . a place where you can retreat at any time. This is a healthy technique for you to learn. . . . This place will help you with your daily stressors.* [If the client is in the hospital, . . .] *This safe and special place is very important, particularly while you are in the hospital. . . . Any time that there are interruptions, just let yourself go to this place in your mind.*
- *Form a clear image of a pleasant outdoor scene, using all of your senses. . . . Breathe . . . smell the fragrances around you . . . Feel . . . feel the texture of the surface under your feet. Hear . . . hear all the sounds in nature, birds singing, wind blowing. See . . . see all the different sights around as you let yourself turn in a slow circle to get a full view of this special space.* [Include taste, if appropriate.]
- *Let a beam of light, such as the rays of the sun, shine on you for comfort and healing. Allow yourself to experience the warmth and relaxation. Form an image of a meadow. Imagine that you are in the meadow. . . . The meadow is full of beautiful grass and flowers. In the meadow, see yourself sitting by a stream . . . watching the water . . . flowing by . . . slowly and gently.*
- *Imagine a mountain scene. See yourself walking on a path toward the mountain. You hear the sound of your shoes on the path . . . smell the pine trees and feel the cool breeze as*

you approach your campsite. You have now reached the foothills of the mountain. You are now higher up the mountain . . . resting in your campsite. Look around at the beauty of this place.

- *Imagine yourself in a bamboo forest. . . . You are walking in a large bamboo forest. The bamboo is very tall. . . . You lean against a strong cluster of bamboo . . . hear the swaying . . . and hear the rustling of the bamboo leaves, gently moving in the wind. . . . Look into the sky of your mind. . . . See the fluffy clouds. A cloud gently comes your way, . . . and the cloud surrounds your body. You climb up on the cloud and lie down. Feel yourself begin to float off gently in a gentle breeze.*

Pain Assessment Imagery.   Imagery helps access and control both acute and chronic psychophysiologic pain. The following exercise can be done in 10 to 20 minutes.

Script: *Close your eyes and let yourself relax. . . . Begin to describe the pain in silence to yourself. Be present with the pain. . . . Know that the pain may be either physical sensations . . . or worries and fears. Let the pain take on a shape . . . any shape that comes to your mind. Become aware of the dimensions of the pain. . . . What is the height of the pain? . . . The width of the pain? . . . And the depth of the pain? Where in the body is it located? . . . Give it color . . . a shape. . . . Feel the texture. Does it make any sound?*

And now with your eyes still closed, . . . let your hands come together with palms turned upward as if forming a cup. Put your pain object in your hands. [Once again, the nurse asks these questions about the pain, preceding each question with this phrase, "How would you change the size, etc.?"]

Let yourself decide what you would like to do with the pain. There is no right way to finish the experience. . . . Just accept what feels right to you. You can throw the pain away . . . or place it back where you found it . . . or move it somewhere else. Let yourself become aware . . . of how pain can be changed. . . . By your focusing with intention, the pain changes.

It is not unusual for the pain to go completely away, or at least lessen after this exercise. The client also learns to manipulate the pain so that it is not the controlling factor of his or her life. The exercise is also effective with severe pain. After giving pain medication, the nurse can have the client relax during the imagery process.

Evaluation

With the client, the nurse determines whether the client outcomes for imagery were successful (Exhibit 22–1). To evaluate the session further, the nurse may again explore the subjective effects of the experience with the client (see Exhibit 22–2).

Imagery is a tool for connecting with the unlimited capabilities of the bodymind. It is a nonverbal modality and a rich resource for information about all life processes. Using imagery, a nurse can help a client make changes in perceptions, behaviors, and attitudes that can promote healing.

Nurse Healer Reflections

- How do I feel about my imagination?
- When I work with imagery, what inner resources can assist me in my life processes?

Exhibit 22-2 Evaluating the Client's Subjective Experience with Imagery

1. Was this a new kind of imagery experience for you? Can you describe it?

2. Did you have a visual experience? Of people, places, or objects? Can you describe them?

3. Did you see colors while being guided? Did the colors change as the guided imagery continued?

4. Were you aware of your surroundings? Were you able to let the imagery flow?

5. Did you like the imagery?

6. Did the imagery produce any feelings or emotions?

7. Did you notice any textures, smells, movements, or tastes while experiencing the imagery?

8. Was the experience pleasant?

9. Did you feel relaxed and refreshed after the experience?

10. Would you like to try this again?

11. What would make this a better experience for you?

12. What is your next step (or your plan) to integrate this on a daily basis?

Notes

1. J. Achterberg, *Imagery in Healing* (Boston: Shambhala, 1985).
2. A.A. Sheikh et al., Healing Images: Historical Perspective, in *Healing Images: The Role of Imagination in Health*, ed. A.A. Sheikh (Amityville, New York: Baywood Publishing Company, Inc., 2003), 3–26.
3. B.G. Schaub and R. Schaub, *Dante's Path: A Practical Approach to Achieving Inner Wisdom* (New York: Gotham Books, 2003).
4. Ibid.
5. J. Achterberg et al., *Rituals of Healing* (New York: Bantam Books, 1994).

CHAPTER 23

Music Therapy: Hearing the Melody of the Soul*

Nurse Healer Objective

- Explore each step of the holistic caring process when using music therapy with various clients to facilitate the healing process.

Definitions

Music Therapy: the behavioral science concerned with the systematic application of music to produce relaxation and desired changes in emotions, behavior, and physiology.

Sound: that which is produced when some object is vibrating in a random or periodic repeated motion.

Holistic Caring Process

Assessment

In preparing to use music therapy interventions, the nurse assesses the following parameters:

- the client's music history and the types of music that the client prefers (Table 23–1)
- the client's ability to identify types of music that make him or her happy, excited, sad, or relaxed (Figure 23–1)
- the client's ability to identify types of music that are distasteful and make him or her tense

---

* Condensed from: C.E. Guzzetta, Music Therapy: Hearing the Melody of the Soul, in *Holistic Nursing: A Handbook for Practice*, 4th ed., eds. B.M. Dossey, L. Keegan, C.E. Guzzetta (Sudbury, MA: Jones and Bartlett Publishers, 2005), 617–640.

Table 23-1 Categories of Music

Category	Composer Sources
Classical Music	Beethoven, Mozart, Haydn, Bach, Dvorak
Baroque Music	Bach, Handel, Vivaldi, Purcell, Pachelbel
Romantic Music	Strauss, Wagner, Schubert, Schumann, Tchaikovsky, Chopin, Liszt, Brahms
Impressionist Music	Debussy, Faure, Ravel, Elgar
Big Band Music	Goodman, Ellington, Dorsey, Lombardo, Miller
Jazz	Davis, Neville, Coltrane, Najee, Koz, James
Blues	John Lee Hooker, Taylor, Cray, Lavette
Country Western	Cash, Nelson
Nontraditional, New Age Music	Halpern, Eno

- the client's awareness of the importance of music in his or her life
- the client's previous participation in relaxation/imagery techniques combined with music: How long? How regularly?
- the client's insight into the use of music to produce psychophysiologic alterations
- the client's mood (iso-principle) that will determine the type of music to choose and the goals of the session

(Assessment parameters outlined in Chapter 21, Relaxation, and Chapter 22, Imagery, also should be included, because relaxation, imagery, and music cannot be separated.)

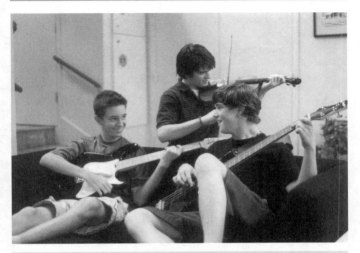

Figure 23-1 Melodic Memories. Courtesy of Philip C. Guzzetta III.

Patterns/Challenges/Needs

The following are the patterns/challenges/needs compatible with music therapy interventions that are related to the 13 domains of Taxonomy II (see Chapter 14):

- Social isolation
- Loneliness
- Spiritual distress
- Ineffective individual coping
- Impaired adjustment
- Noncompliance
- Sleep pattern disturbance
- Sleep deprivation
- Fatigue
- Adult failure to thrive
- Disorganized infant behavior
- Body image disturbance
- Self-esteem disturbance
- Hopelessness
- Powerlessness
- Confusion

- Altered thought
  processes
- Impaired memory
- Pain
- Nausea
- Chronic sorrow

- Risk for violence
- Post-trauma
  syndrome
- Anxiety
- Death anxiety
- Fear

Outcomes

Exhibit 23–1 guides the nurse in client outcomes, nursing prescriptions, and evaluation for the use of music therapy as a nursing intervention.

Therapeutic Care Plan and Implementation

BEFORE THE SESSION

- Inform others of the need for minimal noise.
- Establish the goals for the session with the client.
- Discuss how music therapy quiets the bodymind and facilitates relaxation and self-healing.
- Discuss the length of the session, usually 20 to 30 minutes.
- Ask the client to empty his or her bladder, if necessary.
- Ask the client to remove eyeglasses.
- Prepare the environment for optimal relaxation:
  — Close the drapes.
  — Dim the lights.
  — Turn off any potential environmental noises.
- Ask the client to sit or lie in a comfortable position.
- Spend a few moments centering yourself to be fully present with the client.

AT THE BEGINNING OF THE SESSION

> **Script:** *The purpose of the session is to relax in a wakeful state and have a quiet experience listening to music. First, I*

Exhibit 23-1 Nursing Interventions: Music Therapy

Client Outcomes	Nursing Prescriptions	Evaluation
The client will demonstrate positive physiologic outcomes in response to the music therapy session, such as: • decreased respiratory rate • decreased heart rate • decreased blood pressure • decreased muscle tension • decreased fatigue	Assess the client's psychologic outcomes in response to music therapy before and immediately after the session. Evaluate the client's: • respiratory rate • heart rate • blood pressure • muscle tension • level of fatigue	The client demonstrated: • decreased respiratory rate • decreased heart rate • decreased blood pressure • decreased muscle tension • decreased fatigue
The client will demonstrate positive psychologic outcomes in response to the music therapy: • positive emotions • decreased restlessness • decreased anxiety/depression • increased motivation • increased positive imagery	Assess the client's psychologic outcomes. Evaluate: • emotions • level of restlessness • level of anxiety/depression • level of motivation • type of imagery experienced	The client demonstrated or verbalized: • positive emotions • reduced restlessness • decreased levels of anxiety • increased motivation to accomplish life's daily tasks • increased positive imagery

> will guide you in a few exercises to relax. Then I will
> guide you in how to listen to music (of your choice).
> Then try to let the music relax your body-mind-spirit
> even more as you listen to the music for 20 minutes.
> Now close your eyes if you wish. Find a comfortable
> position with your hands at the side of your chest or on
> your body—whatever is most comfortable. At any
> time, you may change positions, scratch, or swallow.
> There may be noises around, but these will not be
> important if you concentrate on my voice.

Guide the client in a general relaxation or imagery script (see
Chapters 21 and 22).

DURING THE SESSION

Script: Now, as you continue to relax, I will turn on the
music. Listen to the music. Tell yourself that you would
like to go wherever the music takes you. Allow yourself
to follow the music. Let the music suggest to you what
to think and what to feel. Do not try to analyze the
music or the melody. If you find distracting thoughts
occurring, simply let go of them and come back to concentrating on the music. Allow the music to relax you
even more than you are now. The music will play for
20 minutes, and I will leave the room. I will quietly
come back into the room before the music is over. Now
continue to relax your body-mind-spirit; let the music
help you.

AT THE END OF THE SESSION

Script: Now that the music is over, I will guide you in counting
back from 5 to 1. You will come back into the room
easily and quietly. You will feel very relaxed, calm, and
peaceful. You will remember the pathway that led you

> *to this new experience, and you will be able to find it*
> *quickly whenever you wish to return.*

Close the session as follows:

- While the client is in a self-reflective state, lead him or her in further guided imagery exercises, or journal entries, if desired.
- Use the client outcomes (see Exhibit 23–1) that were established before the session and the client's subjective experience (Exhibit 23–2) to evaluate the session.
- Schedule a follow-up session.

Specific Interventions

DEVELOPMENT OF AUDIOCASSETTE/CD/VIDEOCASSETTE LIBRARY

Nurses can develop an audiocassette/CD/videocassette library on each clinical unit or in each practice area. Audiocassettes, CDs, and videocassettes can be developed and collected that are of specific benefit to the particular client/patient population with which the nurse is working. Following are suggestions for building a successful audiocassette/CD/videocassette library:

1. Equipment
   - Have several tape/CD players with comfortable headsets per unit.
   - Place all equipment in a safe and convenient location.
   - Establish a method of headset disinfection to be done after each patient finishes with the equipment.
   - Have a variety of music tapes/CDs available. A complete tape library will include music, relaxation, imagery, and stress management tapes/CDs. Consider different types of music, such as easy listening, light and heavy classical, popular, jazz (see Table 23–1).
   - Ask staff members to donate one favorite relaxation tape/CD to the library.

Exhibit 23-2   Evaluating the Client's Subjective Experience with Music Therapy

1. Was this a new kind of music listening experience for you? Can you describe it?
2. Did you have any visual experiences? Of people, places, or objects? Can you describe them?
3. Did you see any colors while listening? Did the colors change as the music changed?
4. Did you notice any textures, smells, movements, or tastes while experiencing the music?
5. Were you less aware of your surroundings? Were you able to flow with the music?
6. Did you like the music?
7. Did the music produce any feelings or emotions?
8. Was the experience pleasant?
9. Did you feel relaxed and refreshed after the experience?
10. Would you like to try this again?
11. What would be helpful to make this a better experience for you?

- Have brochures and catalogues of recording companies available upon request from the patient.
- Encourage use of different tapes/CDs for further relaxation, imagery, and stress management training.
2. Procedures
   - If tapes/CDs are checked out, have the client make a deposit to cover the replacement cost if not returned.
   - Label all equipment and materials with owner's name, telephone number, and return address.
   - Prepare a sign-out log that records the patient's name, room, date, and check-out time for inpatients or address and telephone number for outpatients.

- Instruct the patient in the use of the equipment and tapes, if necessary.
- Allow 20 to 30 minutes of listening without interruption twice a day.
- Following the listening session, evaluate the patient's response to the music and answer any questions.
- Chart the type of music selected and the patient's specific response to the therapy. Identify the client's subjective evaluation of the experience.
- Return the equipment and tapes/CDs to the library and record the check-in information in the log.

Evaluation

With the client, the nurse determines whether the client outcomes of music therapy (see Exhibit 23–1) were achieved successfully. To evaluate the session further, the nurse may again explore the subjective effects of the experience with the client (Exhibit 23–2).

Nurse Healer Reflections

- How do I feel about music as a healing ritual?
- Am I able to use music with my clients to facilitate the healing process?

Using Our Healing Hands*

Nurse Healer Objective

- Explore each step of the holistic caring process when using touch to connect with the healing power.

Definitions

Acupressure: the application of finger and/or thumb pressure to specific sites along the body's energy meridians for the purpose of relieving tension, reestablishing the flow of energy along the meridian lines, and restoring balance to the human energy system.

Body Therapy and/or Touch Therapy: the broad range of techniques that a practitioner uses in which the hands are on or near the body to assist the recipient toward optimal function.

Caring Touch: touch performed with a genuine interest in the other person, as well as an expression of empathy and concern.

Centering: a sense of self-relatedness that can be thought of as a place of inner being, a place of quietude within oneself where one can feel truly integrated, unified, and focused.

Grounding: the process of connecting to the earth and the earth's energy field, to calm the mind and focus one's inner flow of energy as a means to enhance healing endeavors.

* Condensed from: L. Keegan and K.H. Shames, Using Our Healing Hands, in *Holistic Nursing: A Handbook for Practice*, 4th ed., eds. B.M. Dossey, L. Keegan, C.E. Guzzetta (Sudbury, MA: Jones and Bartlett Publishers, 2005), 643–666.

Intention: the motivation or reason for touching; the direction of one's inner awareness and focus for healing; the state of being fully present in the moment.

Procedural Touch: touch performed to diagnose, monitor, or treat an illness; touch that focuses on the end result of curing the illness or preventing further complications.

Therapeutic Massage: the use of the hands to apply pressure and motion to the recipient's skin and underlying muscle to promote physical and psychologic relaxation, improve circulation, relieve sore muscles, and accomplish other therapeutic effects.

Therapeutic Touch: a specific technique of centering intention used while the practitioner moves the hands through a recipient's energy field for the purpose of assessing and treating energy field imbalance.

Holistic Caring Process

Assessment

In preparing to use touch interventions, the nurse assesses the following parameters:

- the client's perception of his or her bodymind situation.
- the client's potential pathophysiologic problems that may require referral to a physician for evaluation.
- the client's history of psychiatric disorders. The nurse must modify the approach with clients who have present or past psychiatric disorders. Touch itself may present a problem, and the deeply relaxed, semihypnotic state that a balanced person finds enjoyable may actually frighten or alarm an unbalanced individual.
- the client's cultural beliefs and values about touch.
- the client's past experience with body therapies. The knowledge level of clients varies widely. The approach will differ markedly depending on the client's previous experience. Assisting a client in transferring prior learn-

ing, such as from childbirth preparation classes to a new situation, is a valuable nursing intervention.

Patterns/Challenges/Needs

The following are the patterns/challenges/needs compatible with the interventions for touch that are related to the 13 domains of Taxonomy II (see Chapter 14):

- Altered circulation
- Impairment in skin integrity
- Social isolation
- Altered spiritual state
- Impaired physical mobility
- Altered meaningfulness
- Altered comfort
  - Anxiety
  - Grieving
  - Fear

Outcomes

Exhibit 24–1 guides the nurse in client outcomes, nursing prescriptions, and evaluation for the use of touch as a nursing intervention.

Therapeutic Care Plan and Interventions

BEFORE THE SESSION

- Wash your hands.
- Wear loose-fitting, comfortable clothing. If you're wearing street clothes, cover them with a laboratory coat.
- Have the client empty the bladder for comfort.
- Prepare the hospital bed, therapy table, or surface on which you will be working. If you will be using a therapy table, drape it with a cotton blanket and place a sheet over the top. Lay out a large towel for the client to use as a cover when he or she lies on the table. Adjust the height of the table or bed for optimal use of your body mechanics.

Exhibit 24-1   Nursing Interventions: Touch

Client Outcomes	Nursing Prescriptions	Evaluation
The client is relaxed following a touch therapy session.	Encourage the client to receive touch therapy in order to evoke the relaxation response. During the touch therapy session, help the client • decrease anxiety and fear • decrease pulse and respiratory rate • recognize a feeling of body-mind relaxation • develop a sense of general well-being • increase effectiveness in individual coping skills • increase a sense of belonging and lessened loneliness • feel less alone and express that feeling	The client willingly accepted touch therapy. The client • exhibited decreased anxiety and fear • demonstrated a decrease in pulse and respiratory rate • reported muscle relaxation • exhibited satisfied facial expression and expressed inner calmness • reported greater satisfaction in individual coping patterns

The client has improved circulation.	Provide the client with information about how touch therapies improve circulation and tissue perfusion	Clients with white skin had a reddened color in the area where the nurse had used effleurage and pétrissage massage strokes. Skin in the massaged area is warmer than before the therapy.
The client receives touch therapy to maintain and enhance health.	Encourage the client to ask for touch therapy. Suggest that the client seek out the nurse. Recommend that the client accept touch when offered by the nurse.	The client asked for touch therapy.

- Have small pillows or towel rolls available for supporting the head, back, or lower legs.
- Control the room environment so that the room is warm, dimly lit, and quiet. If you are in a client's hospital room, draw the curtain and turn off the television set. A radio or audiocassette player may be left on for soothing music.
- Use relaxation and breathing techniques, imagery, or music to elicit the relaxation response.
- After you have talked with the client, spend a few moments to quiet and center yourself, focus on your healing intention, and then begin.

AT THE BEGINNING OF THE SESSION

- Explain to the client the steps in the touch process to be used. The first session always takes the most time because of the necessary explanations and adjustments. The remaining sessions may last from 15 to 60 minutes.
- As you progress through the intervention, explain what you are about to do before you actually begin. Encourage the client to address concerns or discomfort at any time.
- Position the head comfortably. If the client has long hair, pull it up and away from the neckline.
- If you are working on the client's entire body, have the client disrobe completely and cover up with a towel from the chest to the thighs. The client lies on a padded therapy table or hospital bed that is covered with a cotton blanket and sheet. The sides of the sheet and blanket are then wrapped over the client so that he or she feels protected and warm. (This procedure is used for physical touch therapies and is not needed for Therapeutic Touch or other energy-based interventions, which may be done with the client fully clothed. However, remember that

when the client experiences the relaxation response, the body may undergo cooling.)

- Uncover only the body area that is being massaged or pressed as the therapy proceeds.
- In most cases, begin with the client lying on the back. When therapy on the medial aspect and limbs of the body is complete, lift the wraps and reapply them after the client turns over.
- Encourage the client to take slow, deep, releasing breaths. When he or she lets go of tension through breath, affirm in a soft tone, "Ah, feel the body as it relaxes."
- During the turning process, slide the towel around the client's body to ensure that the client will not be exposed. As the client lies prone, continue the therapy on the dorsal aspect of the body.

DURING THE SESSION

- Be attuned to the client's responses to therapy. This will help the client build trust and achieve optimal relaxation.
- In initial sessions, continue to explain what the client can expect to happen so that he or she feels comfortable with the continued direction of the touch sessions. After trust has been established and the relaxation response is learned, the client will relax more quickly and move to deeper levels in subsequent sessions.
- In subsequent sessions, proceed the same as in the initial session. Explanations may be shorter, however.
- Remember to use your voice in a soft, soothing manner that enables the client to relax.
- Reassess the client's responses as you proceed.

AT THE END OF THE SESSION

- When you have finished the touch therapy session, verbally let the client know that it is time to return gradually to the here and now, to begin to move around slowly, and to awaken fully.

- Anticipate that the client will take a few minutes to re-orient to time and place after being in a deep state of relaxation.
- Allow a period of silence for the client to appreciate fully the wisdom of his or her relaxed bodymind.
- Stay in the room while the client rouses and sits up. Give necessary assistance to ensure a safe transfer to an ambulatory position.
- Allow time to receive the client's verbal feedback about the meaning of the session if the client feels the need to talk. If this does not occur spontaneously, ask for feedback. The insight gained provides guidelines for further sessions or specific ideas that the client can follow up in daily life.
- When the touch therapy is used for relaxation or sleep induction for hospitalized patients, close the session by softly pulling the bedcovers up over the patient's back and quietly turning off the light as the patient moves into sleep. Let the client know in advance that you will leave quietly at the end.
- Use the client outcomes that were established before the session (see Exhibit 24–1) and the client's subjective experience (Exhibit 24–2) to evaluate the session.
- Schedule a follow-up session.

Specific Interventions: Touch

GENERAL TOUCH (BASIC)

Each of the therapies discussed in the text has basic, intermediate, and advanced levels. The complexity of each type depends on the amount of time spent studying the multiple variations of the therapy and whether the therapy is used in conjunction with another therapy, such as music and imagery.

Exhibit 24-2   Evaluation of the Client's Subjective Experience of Touch Therapies

1. Was this a new kind of experience for you? Can you describe it?

2. Did this feel like a comforting, stimulating, or both tactile sensation?

3. Was it pleasurable on all planes—physical, mental, emotional, and spiritual—or more focused in one area than another?

4. Were you aware of your surroundings during the experience, or did you sink into a sense of timelessness?

5. Did emotions surface during the experience? If so, what were they? Can you focus on them now?

6. Did you experience any imagery during the touch session?

7. Did you feel comfortable with the therapist? Is there anything that you want to do to increase your comfort level with the touch therapist?

8. Did you feel relaxed and refreshed after the experience?

9. Would you like to try this again?

10. What would be helpful to make this a better experience for you?

11. Can you develop a plan or strategy to integrate more of the touch therapies into your life on a regular basis?

THERAPEUTIC MASSAGE (BASIC TO ADVANCED)

Although they may be called by different names (massage, Swedish massage, massage therapy), the techniques of therapeutic massage are all essentially the same. They involve the use of effleurage, pétrissage, and tapotement: the classic nursing back-rub strokes. These strokes are designed to enhance the circulation of both blood and lymph. Therapeutic massage increases the dispersion of nutrients to promote the removal of metabolic wastes by increasing both lymphatic and blood flow.

THERAPEUTIC TOUCH (ADVANCED)

Therapeutic Touch is generally taught by experienced practitioners in continuing education seminars. The courses include discussion of some or all of the following elements: centering; assessment; hand scanning; intuition; energy field reading, mapping, and recording; pattern comparison; verbal communication of information; stress levels; relaxation levels; meditation experience.

HEALING TOUCH (ADVANCED)

An energy-based therapeutic approach, healing touch combines philosophy with a way of caring and considers healing a sacred art. It uses a collection of noninvasive, energy-based treatment modalities with the purpose of restoring wholeness through harmony and balance.

ACUPRESSURE AND SHIATZU (BASIC TO ADVANCED)

A broad range and depth of techniques are used in acupressure and Shiatzu. Most practitioners receive continuing education in this area; some spend years perfecting these techniques.

REFLEXOLOGY (BASIC TO ADVANCED)

The primary purpose of reflexology is to evoke bodymind relaxation. When a therapist works on these specific areas, a corresponding energy release or relaxation occurs in the internal body system.

Evaluation

With the client, the nurse determines whether the client outcomes for touch therapies (see Exhibit 24–1) were successfully achieved. To evaluate the session further, the nurse may again explore the subjective effects of the experience with the client using the evaluation questions in Exhibit 24–2.

Nurse Healer Reflections

- How do I feel about using touch as an intervention?
- What do I experience with touch therapy when I touch a client from a place of centeredness?
- When I touch with intention, what is my inner experience?
- When I use touch, what happens to my sense of time?
- How does my touch as a nurse affect the recipient?
- Whom do I know who can be my mentor to help me increase skills with touch?
- What other modalities can be used concurrently to heighten the effectiveness of touch?

Relationships*

Nurse Healer Objective
- Explore each step of the holistic caring process when considering the importance of relationships.

Definitions

Archetype: name given by Jung for specific patterns of human collective awareness that symbolically represent human potentials, such as the Healer, the Warrior, the Mother, or the Wise Person.[1]

Complementary Transaction: an interaction in which the ego states match (e.g., Adult-to-Adult communication). Complementary transactions support and strengthen relationships.

Defense Patterns: protective mechanisms that justify individual action while detracting from relationship building.

Ego State: an identifiable, understandable part of ourselves that is within our conscious awareness. Berne identified at least five ego states that can be brought into awareness for personal change or conflict resolution.[2]

Emotional Intelligence: awareness and attention to personal emotional needs that allow us to be in a position of equality with others, rather than seeking power and control or becoming overly passive.

---

* Condensed from: D. Hover-Kramer, Relationships, in *Holistic Nursing: A Handbook for Practice*, 4th ed., eds. B.M. Dossey, L. Keegan, C.E. Guzzetta (Sudbury, MA: Jones and Bartlett Publishers, 2005), 669–690.

Forgiveness: a willingness to acknowledge one's own mistakes and shortcomings and to allow others room to acknowledge their shortcomings as well.

Game: in psychological terms, a dysfunctional pattern of relationship interaction that is recurring and ends in an emotional payoff or sense of entrapment.[3]

Intimacy: a relationship of deep trust and ability to share oneself fully. Such a relationship may be inappropriate in co-worker and policy-setting environments.

Relationship: a healthy sense of connection in which two or more persons agree to share successes, hurts, failures, learning, in a nonjudgmental fashion to enhance each other's life potentials. In the context of professional settings, healthy relatedness encompasses advocacy, influence, and effective assertiveness.

Uncomplementary Transaction: an interaction in which ego states do not match (e.g., critical Parent-to-Adaptive Child communication) that may lead to the formation of a psychological game; an interaction that reduces relationship formation.

Holistic Caring Process

Assessment

In preparing to use relationship interventions, the nurse can assess the following parameters:

- the ego state most in evidence in the other person's transactions
- the ego state that the nurse is using
- the events that happen repeatedly that may be patterns of a game
- the nurse's feelings (e.g., What is the Child part saying?)
- the nurse's values (e.g., What is the Parent input?)

- the nurse's options (e.g., What is the Adult input?)
- respect for self and the other person
- use of effective assertiveness rather than exerting control or being passive
- opportunities for mutuality in this exchange

Patterns/Challenges/Needs

The following patterns/challenges/needs compatible with the interventions for relationships are associated with the 13 domains of Taxonomy II (see Chapter 14):

- Withdrawal
- Denial
- Repression
- Rationalization
- Regression
- Changes in parenting and family structure
- Human sexual dysfunction
- Lack of social coherence
- Spiritual disconnectedness and distress
- Altered family process
- Ineffective coping
- Self-care deficits
- Self-care dysfunction
- Anxiety
- Grief
- Fear
- Response to trauma

Outcomes

Exhibit 25–1 guides the nurse in client outcomes, nursing prescriptions, and evaluation for using relationships as a nursing intervention.

Exhibit 25-1 Nursing Interventions: *Relationships*

Client Outcomes	Nursing Prescriptions	Evaluation
The client will recognize personal and relationship patterns and how they support or detract from quality of life.	Assist the client in identifying • the importance of relationships • the patterns that increase comfort and effective communication • family relationship patterns and areas that could be improved • sources of emotional stress in his or her relationships • the human needs that are fulfilled by quality relationships • the impact of relationships on health and illness	The client verbalized the dynamics within the family relationship patterns. The client stated the importance of his or her relationships to quality of life. The client identified areas in which relationships could be improved. The client recognized factors that create stressors in relationships. The client stated understanding of the interconnection between relationships and health or illness.
The client will recognize and identify complementary and uncomplementary	Demonstrate examples of complementary and uncomplementary	The client identified a complementary transaction and an uncomplementary transaction.

transactions in relationships.	transactions, and help the client to identify such transactions in family and caregiver relationships.	
The client will increase awareness of Parent, Adult, and Child ego states.	Demonstrate examples of the differences in the three ego states.	The client identified his or her personal use of Parent, Adult, and Child ego states.
The client will identify personal response patterns to others' ego states.	Assist the client in identifying personal response patterns to others' ego states, and help the client to improve the effective expression of inner feelings.	The client recognized another person's use of an ego state and his or her personal response.
	Describe the four archetypes and their applications in communicating physical, emotional, mental, and spiritual perspectives.	
The client will incorporate new strategies to improve the quality of interpersonal	Provide the client with techniques to improve relationships, such as making "I" statements ("This is	The client showed interest in the four archetype patterns and willingness to try out new

(*continues*)

Exhibit 25-1 (continued)

Client Outcomes	Nursing Prescriptions	Evaluation
relationships.	how I feel, . . . My feeling is . . ."), noting ego states in a transaction, and activating the four archetypes.	communications from each perspective.
The client will increase awareness of the physical, emotional, mental, and spiritual aspects of relationship interactions.	Teach the client to express awareness of physical needs and take responsibility for practical aspects of his or her care, such as need for more information and understanding of optimal outcomes.	The client demonstrated the ability to express personal feelings using "I" statements.
The client will recognize opportunities for effective negotiations with willingness to reconsider ineffective aspects.	Assist client to identify arenas where he or she can negotiate, make choices, or reconsider previous decisions; to see the open-ended nature of present relationships, especially with caregivers and family; to view the present disease as an opportunity for learning and change.	The client negotiated effectively after considering options. The client reconsidered relationship interactions that were ineffective. The client expressed interest in the open-ended nature of learning from his or her illness and treatment.

Therapeutic Care Plan and Implementation

BEFORE THE SESSION

- Take a moment to set your intent and focus, allowing yourself to breathe fully, to sense your center, and to align with your sense of purpose.
  — Take several deep breaths and relax the body.
  — Rehearse a new pattern, such as giving accurate facts, in your mind.
  — Imagine the successful outcome.
  — Acknowledge your positive intent.
  — Be willing to learn from each experience.

DURING THE SESSION

- Notice the ego states that are in evidence, specifically the feelings that are triggered within yourself.
- Be aware of ways that finding common ground enhances rapport.
- Consider options that can achieve the goal of the communication.
- Make "I" statements when speaking about your personal point of view or experience.
- Set limits, by determining time frames, topics to be discussed, the context, and the environment.
- Be willing to change direction, or reconsider a point, to come to feasible compromises.
- Above all, keep the intent of the communication positive and maintain a relationship of mutual respect, even though specific content areas may be questioned and differing viewpoints are expressed.

AT THE END OF THE SESSION

- Consider alternatives and make concrete plans for future action.
- Evaluate your own relational skills, your use of different ego states, your use of the archetypes.

- Honor your learning process in accepting mistakes or in thinking about what you might have done differently.
- Consider methods to make trying new behaviors safe and enjoyable, such as sharing your process with a friend or mentor.

Specific Interventions

Counseling.   A client who exhibits normative behavior may seek counseling that focuses on coping behaviors.[4] For example, counseling may involve assistance with smoking cessation or weight reduction. Psychotherapy provides more in-depth interventions, such as working with clients in the struggles and challenges of life roles, individual/family priorities, intimacy, or changing relationship patterns in a marriage. Psychotherapy is definitely indicated when a client exhibits severe personality disorders or pathologic behaviors, although a client need not demonstrate pathology to be referred by the nurse for more in-depth work.

Storytelling.   Stories reveal the importance that we assign to our experiences in life and our perceptions of the world.[5] Storytelling technique becomes advanced when parables and metaphors are used.

Development of Spiritual Understanding.   Individuals must recognize that they are the spiritual experts about their lives, that the journey of wholeness and healing requires spiritual understanding, and that this understanding is a developing process.[6,7]

Facing Fears.   Individuals often have difficulty making changes within relationships or in other life situations because of fear. While there are many different levels of fears—fear of inevitable changes such as those caused by aging or illness, fear of the unknown, fear that we cannot cope with change, fear that we will be alone or abandoned—they have one thing in common: they usually exemplify a concern about something that is not actually occurring in the present moment. Focusing fully on the present is a vitalizing form of relaxation and allows us to manage anticipated distress from a different vantage point.[8]

Improved Communication.   Communication patterns have a direct impact on mind modulation of the autonomic, immune, endocrine, and neuropeptide systems. Because our relationships evoke every conceivable emotion and communication pattern, they have a significant impact on our physiologic state.

Evaluation

With clients or co-workers, the nurse determines whether outcomes for relationship interventions were successfully achieved (see Exhibit 25–1). To evaluate the session or interactions further, the nurse may explore the subjective effects of the experience (Exhibit 25–2).

Conclusion

Inner work with the expressive arts is helpful in understanding personal feelings and clarifying relationship patterns. Ultimately, moving into right relationships with ourselves, each other, and our environment is the healing force for our lives.

Nurse Healer Reflections

- How do I feel at the end of the workday?
- Were there any unpleasant interactions?
- Are there repeated patterns in my relationships that indicate "games" or "payoffs"?
- Will I be able to practice new responses with a friend or co-worker?

Exhibit 25-2   Evaluating the Nurse's Subjective Experience with Relationship Interventions

1. Can you continue to identify and be aware of the relationship that is troublesome to you?
2. Is it possible for you to be clear about your wants and expectations in this relationship?
3. Have you tried out new patterns, such as making a conscious choice of a different ego state? What was the result?
4. Have you considered the transactions in this relationship to make them more complementary?
5. Is it possible for you to communicate your strengths in this relationship? What are the strengths and intent of the other person that could also be acknowledged?
6. Can you imagine how the Healer in you could approach this relationship? How about the Teacher? The Visionary? The practical, grounded Warrior?
7. What would a healed relationship with this person be? How would you feel?
8. Can you identify the steps you could take to move in this direction?
9. What interventions would be most helpful in moving toward healing this relationship?
10. Do you have any questions about any of the new strategies that you have learned for healing this relationship?
11. What is your next step?

Notes

1. C.G. Jung, *Man and His Symbols* (New York: Doubleday & Co., 1964), 67–69.
2. E. Berne, *Principles of Group Treatment* (New York: Oxford University Press, 1964), 281.
3. E. Berne, *Games People Play* (New York: Grove Press, 1964).

4. L. Banks, Counseling, in *Nursing Interventions: Essential Nursing Treatments*, 2nd ed., eds. J. Bulechek and J. McCloskey (Philadelphia: W.B. Saunders, 1992), 279–291.

5. M. Sandelowski, We Are the Stories That We Tell, *Journal of Holistic Nursing* 12, no. 1 (1994):23–33.

6. M. McKivergin and M.J. Daubenmire, The Healing Process of Presence, *Journal of Holistic Nursing* 12, no. 1 (1994):65–81.

7. M. Burkhardt and M.G. Nagai-Jacobson, Reawakening Spirit in Clinical Practice, *Journal of Holistic Nursing* 12, no. 2 (1994): 9–21.

8. D. Hover-Kramer, *Creative Energies: Integrative Psychotherapy for Self-Expression and Healing*, (New York: W.W. Norton, 2002).

CHAPTER 26

Dying in Peace*

Nurse Healer Objective

- Explore each step of the holistic caring process when using dying in peace interventions with clients to facilitate the healing process.

Definitions

Death: a moment in time.

Dying: a stage of life that fits into a broader philosophy, giving both death and life meaning.

Grief: a response to loss, characterized as dynamic, pervasive, individual, yet normative.

Nearing Death Awareness: the dying person's knowledge of death and his or her attempts to describe this experience to health care providers, family, and friends.[1]

Peri-Death: the last hours of life; the actual death and the care of the body after death.[2]

Holistic Caring Process

Assessment

In preparing to use interventions for promoting peaceful dying, the nurse assesses both the dying person and the family or significant others in the following areas:[3,4]

---

* Condensed from: M. Olson, B.M. Dossey, Dying in Peace, in *Holistic Nursing: A Handbook for Practice*, 4th ed., eds. B.M. Dossey, L. Keegan, C.E. Guzzetta (Sudbury, MA: Jones and Bartlett Publishers, 2005), 693–718.

- the different emotions that surface during the process:
  — **guilt:** blame of self and others over management of the dying person; distress over inability to decrease pain.
  — **anger:** toward God, disease, family/significant others, doctors, or survivors; over inability to fix things physically, emotionally, and spiritually.
  — **ability to laugh:** the shortest distance between two people; relationship between comedy and tragedy (joy and sadness pathways cannot operate simultaneously).
  — **love:** an essential element in living and in dying; a state of self-giving and presence of beingness of a person, where openness and willingness exist for self or another; the network that brings and weaves families/significant others together to work through the dying process and move into total acceptance of death.
  — **fear:** often evocation of separateness and aloneness, but can become a path leading deeper into the present moment; useful in that it reveals areas of resistance; return to unconditional love and a sense of equanimity after release of fear.
  — **forgiveness:** an essential element for inner peace; an exercise in compassion that is both a process and an attitude.
  — **faith:** the larger vision of existence, which is different for each person; helps to harness energy to evoke healing resources and power.
  — **hope:** support of patient or family/significant others during death's darkness; an inner moment that perceives lightness when in the midst of darkness and has the potential for leading to deeper love; hope for decreased pain and increased physical and spiritual comfort, for a miracle, for peace of mind, for a remission,

for peaceful death transition, and for acceptance of a shorter life than expected or the death of a loved one.

- the patient's interactions with others and the effect of the patient's emotions on these interactions.
- the need for education about what will happen and what can be done to help, both for the family and the patient.
- comfort needs, assessed according to the patient's culture and wishes.
- assess under- or overmedication that may interfere with a patient's ability to cope with dying.

Patterns/Challenges/Needs

The following are the patterns/challenges/needs compatible with the interventions for dying in peace that are related to the 13 domains of Taxonomy II (see Chapter 14):

- Altered circulation
- Altered oxygenation
- Altered body systems
- Altered communication
- Spiritual distress/well-being
- Ineffective individual/family coping
- Powerlessness
- Hopelessness
- Pain
- Anxiety
- Death anxiety
- Grieving
- Fear

Outcomes

Exhibit 26–1 guides the nurse in identifying patient outcomes, nursing prescriptions, and evaluation for assisting patients and their families/significant others during the dying process.

Exhibit 26-1 Nursing Interventions: Dying in Peace

Patient Outcomes	Nursing Prescriptions	Evaluation
The patient will demonstrate an understanding of reasons for ongoing assessment and management of anxiety.	Continue to reassess states of anxiety and provide ways to decrease anxiety	The patient demonstrated an understanding of the reasons for assessment and management of anxiety.
The patient will verbalize feelings of anxiety and will talk spontaneously about fears. (If the patient is intubated, the patient and the nurse use specific communication codes.)	Provide quality time for the patient to share worries and fears. Use common symbols for communication if the patient is intubated.	The patient verbalized anxiety and fears.
The patient will use effective coping mechanisms during course of illness.	Focus on the patient's strengths.	The patient used effective coping mechanisms during the course of illness. (List specific examples.)
The family will communicate stressors associated with the patient's illness to staff.	Allow time for the family to express worries and fears.	The family/significant others communicated stressors to staff.

(continues)

Exhibit 26-1 (*continued*)

Patient Outcomes	Nursing Prescriptions	Evaluation
The patient will verbalize fears of death.	Be present with the patient and allow time for the patient to talk about fears of dying.	The patient talked of death.
The family/significant others will verbalize fears that the patient may die and what this means to them.	If death seems imminent, be with the patient and family to assist them through the death.	The patient's family/significant others acknowledged the impending death and shared feelings about death.
The family/significant others will receive support from nurses and clergy.	Provide spiritual support for the patient through presence, life review, prayer, talking, and handholding. Allow the family to be with the patient. Call clergy for assistance, if requested.	The family/significant others received spiritual support and talked to nurses and clergy.

Therapeutic Care Plan and Implementation

The following guidelines are appropriate both for the dying person and the caregivers, whether family, friends, or nurse. They are helpful in all settings. The guidelines apply from the first awareness of a coming interaction with a patient and family who are moving through the dying process, through dying, and afterward.

BEFORE THE INTERACTION

- Spend a few moments centering yourself to recognize and honor your presence there.
- Begin the session with intention to facilitate healing and peaceful dying.

AT THE BEGINNING OF THE INTERACTION

- Encourage the patient and the family/significant others as the caregiver(s):
  — set realistic goals.
  — identify different behaviors that have surfaced in their interactions with each other during this period.
  — gather a healing team and honor the patient's personal needs and feelings to avoid more suffering.
  — accept current circumstances, and release things that are beyond their control. Accept the fact that release may not be possible at this time, but they can work toward it.
  — take frequent breaks, at least 20 minutes daily, to evoke quality quiet time with relaxation, imagery, music, meditation, prayer, journal keeping, or dreamwork to assist in the letting-go process.
  — exercise, take long hot baths or showers, eat nutritious foods, eliminate excess caffeine or junk food, and ask other people for relief.
- Encourage the patient and caregivers to tell themselves over and over what a good job they are doing and that

it is the best job that they can do. Repeating it helps in releasing guilt, anger, and frustration.

DURING THE DYING PROCESS

- Recognize the one who is dying as the person who is usually the best teacher about what is right.
- Determine the care needed.
- Explore the advantages and disadvantages of dying at home (or alternative sites).
- Integrate complementary and alternative therapies.
- Recognize the patient's going in and out of awareness. The moment of death itself has no pain, but is a reflex last breath.
- Learn about the changes that occur in the body during dying.
- Understand and accept the body's shutting down.

AT THE MOMENT OF DEATH

- Prepare rituals for the moment of death.
- Surround yourself and the dying person with the peace and the light of love, taking the energy of love and light in with each breath.
- If appropriate, when the person has taken a last breath, carry out additional rituals that may be helpful to those present. Holding hands around the bed, saying a blessing or prayer, or anointing with healing oil, for example, may be planned ahead of time for this moment.
- Schedule a follow-up session/visit with family/significant others, if appropriate. If grief support groups are available, a referral may be helpful.

Specific Interventions

- Incorporate healing rituals with the dying person and the family that may include prayers, mantras, co-

meditation, life review, reading of special poems and sacred text, and death bed rituals.

Relaxation and Imagery Scripts

- Use relaxation and imagery scripts related to letting go,
  opening the heart, forgiving self and others, and releasing grief and pain.

Evaluation

With the patient (family/significant others), the nurse evaluates whether the patient outcomes for planning and implementing a peaceful death (see Exhibit 26–1) were successfully
achieved. To evaluate the interventions further, the nurse may
explore the subjective effects of the experience with the patient (family/significant others), using questions such as those
in Exhibit 26–2.

---

*Exhibit 26–2 Evaluating the Patient's (Family's/Significant
Other's) Subjective Experience with Dying Interventions*

1. Can you continue to be aware of ways to recognize your
   anxiety, fear, and grief at this time?
2. Which of your strengths can best serve you as you move
   through this difficult time?
3. What are the things that you will do to take care of yourself at this time?
4. Do you have any questions that I can help you with just
   now?

Note: These subjective experiences may be used in helping a
patient/family/significant others during the dying process or with the
family/significant others during the grieving process.

Nurse Healer Reflections

- Do I feel a greater sense of healing intention when I include relaxation, imagery, or music in my daily life?

- What are the effects on me when I guide others in healing modalities to facilitate peace in dying?

- How do I know that I am actively listening?

- What new death mythologies and skills can assist me in releasing attachment to my physical body, my possessions, and the people in my life?

Notes

1. M. Callanan and P. Kelly, *Final Gifts: Understanding the Special Awareness, Needs, and Communication of the Dying* (New York: Bantam Books, 1993).

2. M.L. Matzo, Peri-death Nursing Care, in *Palliative Nursing: Quality Care at the End of Life*, eds. M.L. Matzo and D.W. Sherman, (New York: Springer Publishing Co., 2001).

3. M. Olson, *Healing the Dying* (Albany, NY: Delmar Publishers, 1997).

4. ELNEC (End-of-Life Consortium), *Graduate Curriculum: Faculty Guide* (City of Hope & American Association of Colleges of Nursing, 2003).

Weight Management Counseling*

Nurse Healer Objective

- Explore each step of the holistic caring process when using weight management interventions with various clients to facilitate the healing process.

Definitions

Body Mass Index (BMI): weight [kg]/height squared [m²] with healthy weight $\leq$ 24.9.

Obesity: body mass index $\geq$ 30.

Overeating: eating when not hungry or eating more than is required to satisfy hunger.

Overfat: percentage of body fat greater than recommended for a client's gender and age (e.g., 28 percent for women and 20 percent for men).

Overweight: body mass index ranging from 25 to 29.9.

Self-Talk: mental verbalizations that elicit emotional responses.

Weight Cycling/Yo–Yo Dieting: repeated weight loss greater than 10 pounds followed by weight gain three or more times over the past 2 years.

Weight Management: holistic, long-term lifestyle adjustments in clients' bio-psycho-social-spiritual dimensions to promote a high level of individual wellness; caring for and assisting clients to reach sufficient self-acceptance,

---

* Condensed from: S. Popkess-Vawter, Weight Management Counseling, in *Holistic Nursing: A Handbook for Practice*, 4th ed., eds. B.M. Dossey, L. Keegan, C.E. Guzzetta (Sudbury, MA: Jones and Bartlett Publishers, 2005), 721–755.

self-love, and self-responsibility to adjust their lifestyles to support eating for hunger, exercising regularly, and esteem for self and others.

Holistic Caring Process

Assessment

In preparing to use weight management interventions, the nurse assesses the following parameters:

- **body composition**—baseline and at least every 6 months
- **resting heart rate and blood pressure**
- **blood profile**—baseline and at least every 6 months
- **physical fitness**
- **psychological profile**

Patterns/Challenges/Needs

Specific patterns/challenges/needs related to the holistic self-care model and reversal theory include the following:

- Overeating related to increased tension stress.
- Decreased aerobic/resistance exercise related to a poor body image and a feeling of being unworthy to take time for self to exercise.
- Infrequent episodes of play which are related to early modeling and values that consider work to be more important than play.
- Lack of skills to express anger/disagreement related to belief that it is unacceptable behavior.
- Lack of skills to express feelings related to early suppression of feelings as a self-protective mechanism.
- Inability to put self first related to early teaching that others have greater value and worth.

Outcomes

Prochaska and DiClemente developed the transtheoretical therapy model to expand the applicability of change theory.[1]

Their stages of change have been applied to a wide variety of health care problems, including weight management. They proposed that individuals may move through five stages of motivational readiness when confronted with lifestyle changes: (1) precontemplation, (2) contemplation, (3) preparation, (4) action, and (5) maintenance. Nurses should tailor their assessments, interventions, prescriptions, and evaluations to the individual's stage to attain long-term weight management (Exhibit 27–1).

Therapeutic Care Plan and Implementation

BEFORE THE SESSION

- Spend a few moments centering yourself.
- Create an environment in which the client will be encouraged to share his or her story.

AT THE BEGINNING OF THE SESSION

- Show a listing of the stages of change to the client. Accordingly, proceed with the holistic self-care model as shown in Exhibit 27–1.

AT THE END OF THE SESSION

- Ask the client to review what he or she gained from the session and answer any questions. Give the client a copy of any relevant support materials, and ask him or her to explain how to use them. Ask him or her to complete a copy of the weekly calendar and verbalize what he or she has written and the times allotted for the behaviors.

Specific Interventions

Specific interventions used in the holistic self-care model are listed and interpreted according to the five stages of change as described in Exhibit 27–1.[2]

Exhibit 27-1   Nursing Interventions: Long-Term Weight Management According to Prochaska and DiClemente's Stages of Change

Client Outcomes According to Stage of Change	Nursing Prescriptions	Evaluation
Precontemplation (no intention of changing in the next 6 months): The client will verbalize reasons for not wanting to reduce weight and fat, and perform regular exercise.	Measure client's body mass index, body fat, resting heart rate and blood pressure, cholesterol, lipids, and blood glucose. Administer life review and dieting history, BULIT[3] (bulimia test) scale to screen for bulimia, and body image 10-point visual analog scale.	The client received a clinic weight management brochure with written report of her or his physical and psychologic findings. The client verbalized understanding of the report, implied risks, and invitation to learn more about the clinic weight program.
Contemplation (considering changing in the next 6 months, but not active yet): The client will report fewer overeating episodes and less tension stress during daily eating.	Assist the client to apply the EAT for hunger cognitive restructuring nutritional strategy based on reversal theory. Administer Tension Stress Scale.[4]	The client verbalized the three steps of the EAT for Hunger strategy and one difficulty with the strategy to work on in the next 6 months. The client was pleased with freedom of eating for hunger.

Preparation (making some changes, but not at goal): The client will report exercising more frequently, resulting in greater muscle strength, less fatigue, and more energy.	Assist the client to apply the Exercise for LIFE strategy based on reversal theory.	The client described aerobic and strength exercises that she or he is willing to do and one difficulty with the strategy to work on in the next 6 months. The client reported lower tension stress.
Action (6 months of active behavior change): The client will have lower levels of total cholesterol and low-density lipoproteins, a higher level of high-density lipoproteins, and blood glucose levels within normal limits.	Assist the client to apply the STOP Emotional Eating cognitive restructuring psycho-social-spiritual strategy based on reversal theory.	The client verbalized the four steps of the STOP Emotional Eating strategy and one difficulty with the strategy to work on in the next 6 months. The client is pleased with exercise progress.
Maintenance (sustained change past 6 months): The client will have a lower percentage of body fat, lower weight, lower resting heart rate, and lower blood pressure.	Assist the client to apply the acceptance of obstacles cognitive restructuring psycho-social-spiritual strategy.	The client verbalized the acceptance strategy and one difficulty with the strategy on which to concentrate efforts in the next 6 months. The client is pleased with lipid levels, weight, and blood pressure.

PRECONTEMPLATION

When clients are not ready to make lifestyle changes, a nurse cannot "motivate" or manipulate them to do so. The nurse can inform them about his or her assessment of their situation, risks involved, and options available to them.

CONTEMPLATION

Clients in the contemplation stage still believe that the reasons for not changing their behaviors (e.g., I am too tired) over balance the reasons that they should.

EAT for Hunger Strategy.   Under the EAT for Hunger strategy, clients learn to eat according to their internal control (hunger) with as many food choices as desired; regulation of eating is according to internal satiation of their hunger.

Ways to Stop Overeating.   The three steps to stop overeating are written as positive self-talk (affirmations):

1. I eat only when I'm hungry, after rating my hunger on a scale of 1 to 10.
   a. Ravenously starved = 1
   b. Uncomfortably stuffed = 10
   c. Feeling nothing = 5
   d. Eating to satisfy hunger = between 4 and 6
2. I eat exactly what I want. My body has the natural ability to know what it wants and needs.
3. I stop eating when my hunger is gone and I feel nothing (a rating of 5 on the 1 to 10 hunger scale).

PREPARATION

In the preparation stage, clients begin to make lifestyle changes, but they perform the new behaviors sporadically. The Exercise for LIFE strategy is introduced at this stage because individuals often need to be at a higher level of change.

Exercise for LIFE Strategy. The purpose of the Exercise for LIFE strategy is to introduce regular, challenging exercise as a means to express self-value and love. The LIFE stands for Love self In Fitness and Exercise.

ACTION

At six months, clients usually have their eating and exercise habits well under control and have experienced pride and satisfaction in their lifestyle changes. It is especially important at this stage to introduce the cognitive portion of the intervention to help prevent relapse.

STOP Emotional Eating Strategy. The purpose of the STOP Emotional Eating strategy is to separate emotions from eating responses and direct actions for managing underlying stress without eating to cope. Clients can be given copies of books such as *Self-Esteem,*[5] *The Language of Letting Go,*[6] and *Fight Fat After Forty.*[7]

Ways to Change Negative Self-Talk Triggers. Helping clients use reversal theory[8] to balance their ways of being human begins with an examination of the frequent emotions found to trigger overeating and lack of exercise. At this point, the effort focuses on desensitizing, practicing, and accepting being in the negativistic state. Then the four steps for fighting fair are phrased as positive self-talk (affirmations):

1. I tell objectively the facts about what happened. ("I saw you with Lucy after you told me you didn't have time to get together this evening.")
2. I tell what I didn't like about his or her behavior. ("I didn't like seeing you with another of your friends after you told me you didn't have time for us to get together.")
3. I tell how I feel about it. ("I felt pushed aside for you to be with Lucy instead of me; I felt unimportant; I felt lonely.")

4. I tell what I realistically want him or her to do. ("I would like to spend time with you every week, and I would like you to make some time for me if that's what you want also.")

By knowing the positive and negative feelings, clients can pinpoint states in which they repeatedly experience increased tension stress and turn to overeating to deal with the unpleasant feelings.[9]

MAINTENANCE

Beyond six months of clients' practicing and refining lifestyle changes, the nurse can be very instrumental in helping them maintain their lifestyle changes by continuing supportive actions. The final key to lasting change is *acceptance*. When clients fully accept sadness, anger, and the bad, irritating things in life, rather than try to change perfectly, manipulate, succumb to, and overpower these things, a peace can settle into their spirits. Acceptance opens new possibilities that can help move them ahead to grow beyond obstacles.

Evaluation

With clients, the nurse determines whether their outcomes for weight management were achieved (see Exhibit 27–1). To evaluate clients' progress on goals, the nurse examines with them their weekly and daily calendar sheets. Together, the nurse and a client may explore the subjective effects of their experiences in the program by answering the questions found in Exhibit 27–2.

Nurse Healer Reflections

- How did I accommodate my eating within the food pyramid and the American Diabetic Association diet using the EAT for Hunger strategy?

> *Exhibit 27-2   Evaluating the Client's Subjective Experience with Weight Management Interventions*
>
> 1. How am I feeling about myself and my progress right now?
> 2. Do I have any questions about my eating and exercise programs?
> 3. What new insights have I gained about my self-talk?
> 4. What is my next step, and do I need help to take that step?
> 5. Are my goals realistic for me right now?
> 6. What pain and joy can I expect in reaching my goals?
> 7. Am I seeking my Higher Power to accept the things that I cannot change, and am I thinking positively about changing the things I can change?

- How did my personal aerobic and strength exercise program incorporate the Exercise for LIFE strategy?
- How did I deal directly with unpleasant feelings, instead of eating to cope, using the STOP overeating strategy?

Notes

1. J.O. Prochaska and C.C. DiClemente, In Search of How People Change, *American Psychologist* 47 (1992):1102.
2. B.H. Marcus and L.H. Forsyth, The Challenge of Behavior Change, *Medicine and Health* 80 (1997):300–302.
3. S.A. Popkess-Vawter et al., Use of the BULIT Bulimia Screening Questionnaire To Assess Risk and Progress in Weight Management for Overweight Women Who Weight Cycle, *Addictive Behaviors* 24 (1999):497–507.
4. S.A. Popkess-Vawter et al., Development and Testing of the Tension Stress Scale, *Journal of Nursing Measurement* 8 (2002):2.
5. M. McKay and P. Fanning, *Self-Esteem* (Oakland, CA: New Harbinger Publications, 2000).

6. M. Beattie, *The Language of Letting Go: Daily Medications for Codependents* (New York: Harper Collins, 1990).

7. W. Dyer, *10 Secrets for Success and Inner Peace* (Carlsbad, CA: Hay House, 2001).

8. S.A. Popkess-Vawter et al., Reversal Theory, Overeating, and Weight Cycling, *Western Journal of Nursing Research* 20 (1998): 67–83.

9 S.A. Popkess-Vawter et al., Unpleasant Emotional Triggers to Overeating and Related Intervention Strategies for Overweight and Obese Women Weight Cyclers, *Journal of Applied Nursing Research* 11 (1998):69–76.

Smoking Cessation: Freedom from Risk*

Nurse Healer Objective

- Explore each step of the holistic caring process when using smoking cessation interventions with various clients to facilitate the healing process.

Definitions

Focused Smoking: a smoking reduction technique done under supervision.

Habit Breakers: new action behaviors that replace old smoke signals.

Nicotine Fading: gradual reduction of the nicotine level in the body to avoid withdrawal symptoms.

Holistic Caring Process

Assessment

In preparing to use smoking cessation interventions, the nurse assesses the following parameters:

- the client's level of addiction to cigarettes
- the client's attitudes and beliefs about successful and sustained smoking cessation
- the client's motivation to learn interventions to become a permanent nonsmoker

* Condensed from: C.A. Wynd, B.M. Dossey, Smoking Cessation: Freedom from Risk, in *Holistic Nursing: A Handbook for Practice*, 4th ed., eds. B.M. Dossey, L. Keegan, C.E. Guzzetta (Sudbury, MA: Jones and Bartlett Publishers, 2005), 759–780.

- the client's stage of change in terms of smoking cessation
- the client's eating patterns and exercise program
- the client's existing stress management strategies
- the client's support and encouragement from family and friends

Patterns/Challenges/Needs

The following are patterns/challenges/needs compatible with smoking cessation interventions that are related to the 13 domains of Taxonomy II (see Chapter 14):

- Altered circulation
- Altered oxygenation
- Spiritual distress
- Spiritual well-being
- Ineffective individual coping
- Effective individual coping
- Self-care deficit
- Disturbance in body image
- Disturbance in self-esteem
- Hopelessness
- Knowledge deficit
- Anxiety
- Fear

Outcomes

Exhibit 28–1 guides the nurse in client outcomes, nursing prescriptions, and evaluation for successful smoking cessation.

Therapeutic Care Plan and Implementation

Before the Session

- Spend a few moments centering yourself to recognize your presence and to begin the session with the intention to facilitate healing.
- Gather teaching sheets to be used during the session.
- Create a quiet place to begin guiding the client in smoking cessation strategies.

Exhibit 28-1 Nursing Interventions: Smoking Cessation

Client Outcomes	Nursing Prescriptions	Evaluation
The client will demonstrate attitudes, beliefs, and behaviors that indicate the desire to be a nonsmoker.	Determine the client's desire to be a nonsmoker.	The client demonstrated attitudes, beliefs, behaviors, and the desire to be a nonsmoker.
	Assist the client in setting realistic plans for being a nonsmoker by: • establishing a quit date • drawing up a nicotine withdrawal schedule • cleansing self and environment of nicotine • developing habit-breaker strategies • keeping a smoking diary • practicing relaxation and imagery • integrating behavior changes • deciding on rewards for attaining goals	The client set a realistic plan and became a nonsmoker over 1 week as follows: • focused on quit date goal • went "cold turkey" • cleansed body/environment of nicotine • adhered to habit-breaker strategies • kept a smoking, exercise, food diary • practiced relaxation/imagery daily • integrated behavior changes daily • rewarded self for attaining goals

AT THE BEGINNING OF THE SESSION

- Go over the results of the smoking profile, and explore the meaning of these patterns with the client. Elicit insight into changing behaviors.
- Instruct the client in the importance of keeping a smoking diary.
- Establish pre-quitting strategies. Suggest that the client be patient and identify and combine the methods that can work best.
- Encourage the client to take a few days before the quit date to rid the body of toxins and to clean the house, office, and car of any evidence of cigarettes or odors.
- Have the client establish the quit date and sign a contract that specifies the quit date.
- Encourage the client to call on family and friends on the first smoke-free days, particularly when confidence is low. Remind them that their support is very important.

DURING THE SESSION

- Reinforce the quit date and have the client imagine being smoke-free in five days.
- Teach basic relaxation (see Chapter 21) and imagery (see Chapter 22) skills to shape bodymind changes for internal and external smoke-free images.

    1. Active images—cleansing the body of nicotine and other toxins; finding a safe place that establishes a feeling of security and comfort; envisioning a protective bubble that receives what is needed from others and blocks out negative images, such as smoking triggers.
    2. Process images—people, events, and situations that make the client smoke. Have the client rehearse being in a situation where smoking normally occurs,

but now using a new behavior, such as reaching for a glass of water.

3. End-state images—being smoke-free; accessing one's inner healer.

- Have the client create strategies to break smoking triggers and become smoke-free—waking up and having a glass of water, reading the morning paper in a different room, taking a break and drinking water or juice, talking on the telephone, and practicing relaxation and rhythmic breathing.

AT THE END OF THE SESSION

- Suggest that the client create a personal reward after five smoke-free days.
- Evaluate with the client the goals of behavior changes—reduction of smoking urges and development of new habit patterns.
- Reinforce the fact that the client can avoid relapse. Having learned to recognize high-risk situations for relapse, the client can be ready to act quickly in using strategies to resist smoking temptations.
- Suggest that the client become a support person for someone else who is trying to become smoke-free to decrease chances of relapse.
- Use the client outcomes (see Exhibit 28–1) that were established before the session to evaluate the session.
- Schedule a follow-up session.

Specific Interventions

Stages of Change. Two major constructs organize the framework of the *stages* and the *processes* of change. Five stages of change provide a temporal structure for monitoring the change process. Applied to smoking cessation, the five stages of change are:

1. Precontemplation: no intention of quitting within the next 6 months.
2. Contemplation: seriously considering quitting within the next 6 months.
3. Preparation: seriously planning to quit within the next 30 days and has made at least one quit attempt in past year.
4. Action: former smoker continuously quit for less than 6 months.
5. Maintenance: former smoker continuously quit for greater than 6 months.

The stages are important for measuring progress toward quitting and helping to predict relapse.[1,2]

- *Record smoking habits.*
- *Prepare for quit date.*
- *Preparation for nicotine withdrawal.*   There is no one best way to quit smoking. Some people are successful at just quitting "cold turkey" and going through the nicotine withdrawal, with the worst part usually lasting five days or less. Others require a gradual decrease of nicotine with the use of Nicotine Replacement Therapy (NRT).[3,4] The client must decide which way is best for him or her.
- *Prepare smoke-free body and environment.*   During the first few nonsmoking days, the client rids the body of toxic waste left from the cigarettes by bathing, brushing teeth, drinking water, exercise, relaxation, imagery, rest, and good nutrition. A fresh nonsmoking living environment can be accomplished by placing clean filters in heating and cooling units and cleaning carpets, drapes, clothes, office, and car. Signs may be placed on the office door: "Thank you for not smoking."
- *Identify habit breakers.*   Becoming smoke-free is directly related to minor changes in daily routines, referred to as habit breakers.
- *Integrate exercise.*

- *Use steps to avoid weight gain.*   (see Chapter 27)
- *Integrate rewards.*   The client should plan a reward at least every five to seven days for having a smoke-free lifestyle. These rewards should continue as long as the client needs to be aware of new lifestyle habits. The client is considered smoke-free when his or her habits are indeed nonsmoking behaviors. Continued use of the listed habit breakers always helps a client anticipate when smoke signals can surface and, thus, quickly take actions to prevent relapse.
- *Reinforce positive self-talk.*   Feelings, moods, behaviors, and motivation affect physiologic changes. As the client learns to recognize the self-talk that sabotages his or her positive outlook, it is possible for the client to remain in control and not give in to the urge to smoke.
- *Guide client in smoking cessation imagery scripts.* These scripts are related to quit date, cleansing body and environment of smoke, recognizing smoke triggers, health nutrition, and exercise.

Evaluation

With the client, the nurse determines whether the client outcomes for smoking cessation (see Exhibit 28–1) were achieved. To evaluate the session further, the nurse may again explore the subjective effects of the experience with the client (Exhibit 28–2).

In becoming an ex-smoker, a client must understand that it is a gradual, step-by-step process that requires learning new skills. Smoking cessation involves (1) recognizing smoking habits, (2) establishing habit breakers, (3) preparing for detoxification of body and environment, (4) following a good nutrition and exercise program, and (5) modifying behavior. The integration of these five areas helps clients achieve new awareness about being smoke-free with new lifestyle patterns and improved relationships with people at work and at home.

Exhibit 28–2   Evaluating the Client's Subjective Experience with Smoking Cessation Interventions

1. Did you gain any new insight today about your smoking patterns?
2. Do you have any questions about preparing for a quit date?
3. Do you have any questions about recording your habits?
4. Can you identify two new habit breakers right now to be smoke-free?
5. Are you aware of your bodymind signals of wanting to smoke?
6. What relaxation exercises are most helpful to you in replacing smoking habits?
7. What will be your exercise program?
8. Do you have any questions about the active, process imagery and the end-state imagery exercises that you experienced today?
9. Did you like the imagery exercises?
10. Did you gain any new insight about your self-talk of being smoke-free?
11. What are three affirmations to help you just now create an image change of being smoke-free?
12. What is your next step?

Nurse Healer Reflections

- What rituals can I create or assist others in creating to detoxify and cleanse the body and environment of all traces of nicotine?

Notes

1. J.O. Prochaska et al., In Search of How People Change: Applications to Addictive Behaviors, *American Psychologist* 47, no. 9 (1992):1102.

2. J.O. Prochaska et al., Standardized, Individualized, Interactive and Personalized Self-Help Programs for Smoking Cessation, *Health Psychology* 12 (1993):399–405.

3. J. Stapleton, Commentary: Progress on NRT for smokers, *British Medical Journal* 318 (1999):289.

4. C. Silagy et al., Nicotine Replacement Therapy for Smoking Cessation, *Cochrane Database of Systematic Reviews* 4 (2002), (*http: //www. cochrane.org/cochrane/revabstr/ ab000146.htm.*

CHAPTER 29

Addiction and Recovery Counseling*

Nurse Healer Objective

- Explore each step of the holistic caring process when using addition and recovery counseling interventions with clients to facilitate the healing process.

Definitions

Addiction: a physiological or psychological dependence on a substance (e.g., alcohol, cocaine) or behavior (e.g., gambling, sex, eating).

Denial: a major dynamic in the process of addiction in which the person willfully refuses to accept the reality of his or her behavior and its effect on self and others.

Detoxification: the physical process of withdrawing from use of drugs or alcohol.

Dry Drunk: referring to alcoholism (dry = not drinking) where a person has stopped drinking but has not extended this change to developing mentally, emotionally, and spiritually.

New Consciousness: a concept used in Alcoholics Anonymous that refers to a movement away from addictive thinking and toward an understanding of one's life purpose or spiritual purpose.

---

* Condensed from: B.G. Schaub, B.M. Dossey, Addiction and Recovery Counseling, in *Holistic Nursing: A Handbook for Practice*, 4th ed., eds. B.M. Dossey, L. Keegan, C.E. Guzzetta (Sudbury, MA: Jones and Bartlett Publishers, 2005), 783–810.

Recovery: the mental, emotional, physical, and spiritual actions that support conscious living and freedom from addictive behaviors.

Relapse: a return to addictive behavior, even if on only one occasion.

Spiritual Awakening: an expansion of awareness that results in a realization that the isolated individual is, in fact, participating in a universe of divine intention and order.

Holistic Caring Process

Assessment

In preparing to use strategies to assist clients in overcoming alcoholism, the nurse assesses[1,2]

- the client's characteristics that may suggest alcoholism
  - restlessness, impulsiveness, anxiety
  - selfishness, self-centeredness, lack of consideration
  - stubbornness, irritability, anger, rage, ill humor
  - physical cruelty, brawling, child/spouse abuse
  - depression, isolation, self-destructiveness
  - aggressive sexuality, often accompanied by infidelity, which may give way to sexual disinterest or impotence
  - arrogance that may lead to aggression, coldness, or withdrawal
  - low self-esteem, shame, guilt, remorse, loneliness
  - reduced mental and physical function; eventual blackouts
  - susceptibility to other disease
  - lying, deceit, broken promises
  - denial that there is a drinking problem
  - projection of blame onto people, places, and things
- the client's attitudes, beliefs, and motivation to learn interventions to become nonaddicted
- the client's available family and friends

- the client's eating and exercise patterns
- the client's existing stress management strategies
- the client's willingness to join a support group
- identify early, middle, and late stages of addictive cycle
- the client's specific cycle of addition
- recognize early, middle, and late stage of addictive cycle.[3]

EARLY STAGE OF ADDICTIVE CYCLE

1. unsafe feelings
2. mental focus on the feelings
3. a desire to get rid of the feelings
4. using chemicals to get rid of the feelings
5. nervous system disturbance because of the chemicals
6. unsafe feelings

In the middle stage of addiction, the unsafe feeling is not experienced as a thought. It is experienced only as danger or discomfort. The person knows that immediate relief comes with use of the substance.

MIDDLE STAGE OF ADDICTIVE CYCLE

1. unsafe feeling
2. using chemicals to get rid of the feelings
3. nervous system disturbance because of the chemicals
4. unsafe feelings

LATE STAGE OF ADDICTIVE CYCLE

1. nervous system disturbance
2. using chemicals
3. nervous system disturbance

Patterns/Challenges/Needs

The following are the patterns/challenges/needs compatible with interventions for addictions that are related to the 13 domains of Taxonomy II (see Chapter 14):

- Altered nutrition (more/less than body requirements)
- Altered social interaction
- Altered family processes
- Spiritual distress
- Noncompliance
- Health-seeking behaviors
- Decreased physical mobility
- Sleep pattern disturbance
- Hopelessness
- Powerlessness
- Knowledge deficit
- Anxiety
- Potential for violence
- Fear

Outcomes

Exhibit 29–1 guides the nurse in client outcomes, nursing prescriptions, and evaluation for overcoming addictions.

Therapeutic Care Plan and Implementation

BEFORE THE SESSION

- Spend a few moments centering yourself, connecting with your inner wisdom and intention to facilitate healing.
- Create a quiet place to begin guiding the client in strategies to overcome addiction(s).

AT THE BEGINNING OF THE SESSION

- Review the results of the self-assessment.
- Reinforce the concept that overcoming addictions is a process requiring commitment, new behavioral skills, and support from family and friends.
- Ask the client to tell his or her personal story.
- Assist the client in identifying the steps necessary for overcoming addictions. If necessary, assist the client in going through detoxification.

Exhibit 29-1 Nursing Interventions: Overcoming Addiction

Client Outcomes	Nursing Prescriptions	Evaluation
The client will demonstrate attitudes, beliefs, and behaviors that result in overcoming addictions.	Determine the client's intention to overcome addiction by: • seeking support from healthy family and friends • attending AA meetings • seeking support of a sponsor • detoxifying self and environment of alcohol/drugs • practicing relaxation and imagery • integrating behavioral changes • selecting ways to reward self for attaining goals	The client demonstrated attitudes, beliefs, and actions that reflect an intention to overcome addiction. The client set realistic plans for overcoming addiction as evidenced by: • accepted support of healthy family or friends • attended AA daily • contacted AA sponsor regularly • detoxified self and environment of drugs and alcohol • practiced relaxation/imagery daily • integrated behavioral changes on a daily basis • rewarded self for attaining set goals

DURING THE SESSION

- Teach the client general relaxation and imagery exercises with a focus on awareness of body sensations and their connection to feelings.
- Teach the client how to create specific imagery patterns (see Chapter 22) and to practice and integrate the following:
    1. *active images*—cleansing the body of impurities.
    2. *end-state images*—of feeling healthy, of living with a sense of accomplishment and satisfaction, of having healthy supportive relationships.
    3. *healing images*—connecting with inner healer, inner wisdom, and with spiritual resources.
    4. *process images*—imagining successfully overcoming drink or drug signals and making healthy alternative choices.
- Teach the client to reframe current situations and problems.
- Teach the client to use H.A.L.T., checking to notice if being Hungry, Angry, Lonely, or Tired is a contributing factor when experiencing drink or drug signals. Encourage the client to avoid these conditions whenever possible.
- Encourage the development of creative skills as a means of working with strong emotions and experiences.

AT THE END OF THE SESSION

- Encourage the client to explore the value of a 12-step program as an adjunct to treatment.[3]
- Emphasize the value of selecting someone in the program as a sponsor, so that a support person is available to be contacted on a daily basis.
- Reinforce the idea that the client can outwit relapse by learning how to recognize high-risk situations.

Reinforce the value of using H.A.L.T. when experiencing signals for substance use. Is Hunger, Anger, Loneliness, or Tiredness contributing to these feelings? Encourage the client to make a list of particular high-risk situations and decide in advance quick action steps to prevent relapse.

- Reinforce the importance of integrating healthful habits into daily life. Encourage the client to select one or two practices to which he or she is willing to make a commitment to include in daily life. Imagery, breathing exercises, meditation, yoga, jogging or other physical activities, and dietary changes are all of value.
- Use the client outcomes (see Exhibit 29–1) that were established before the session to evaluate the session.
- Schedule a follow-up session.

Specific Interventions

Support from Family and Friends.   The best gift that a family can give an addicted member is to affirm that the person is loved unconditionally, but that the addicted behavior can no longer be tolerated. *Each family is unique.* The family must decide the best approach to help that member and the whole family with recovery. It is helpful for the spouse to get professional help, as many husbands and wives are blamed—or blame themselves—for a spouse's addiction. Professional counseling for the family is advisable even if the addicted person chooses to join a support group.

Support Groups and Professional Help.   The client needs to continually assess personal and work life stressors. Because group support is vital to success, the client should become actively involved in a local support group for those with his or her specific addiction. Group support programs based on the 12-step programs—for example, Alcoholics Anonymous (AA), Narcotics Anonymous (NA), OverEaters Anonymous

(OA), and CoDependency Anonymous (CODA)—are helpful. These groups are listed under the specific types of addiction in the telephone directory. Alcoholics Anonymous is the best known support program, with a success rate that studies show is on a par with, or better than, expensive inpatient programs. The client also should seek out a professional who is knowledgeable about addictions.

Evaluation

With the client, the nurse determines whether the client outcomes for overcoming addictions (see Exhibit 29–1) were achieved. To evaluate the session further, the nurse may explore the subjective effects of the experience with the client (Exhibit 29–2).

Exhibit 29-2   *Evaluating the Client's Subjective Experience with Overcoming Addictions*

1. What new awarenesses have you had today?
2. Do you understand how to keep a journal of your habits?
3. Can you identify two habit breaker strategies that you are planning to utilize?
4. Are you aware of your bodymind's signals of wanting a drink?
5. Which relaxation exercises are you finding most beneficial?
6. Do you have any questions on how best to practice your imagery and meditation?
7. What physical activities are you including in your daily routine?
8. Have you been monitoring the pattern of your craving by using H.A.L.T.?

9. What affirmations are you working with to reinforce your intentions to be conscious and sober?

10. What have you observed about your patterns of response to vulnerability? Do you tend toward willfulness or willlessness?

11. What have you discovered is your preferred way of connecting with your spiritual nature?

12. What is your next step?

Nurse Healer Reflections

- What addictive patterns do I recognize in my own life?
- What patterns of response to vulnerability do I observe in myself?
- What practices and changes am I willing to bring into my life to encourage my own healing?
- Who are the people in my life who would support me in making healthy changes?
- Can I allow an image to emerge that represents my inner wisdom?
- Can I identify what interferes with my connection to my inner wisdom?
- How do I connect with my spiritual nature and how do I support this in my daily life?

Notes

1. B. Schaub and R. Schaub, *Healing Addictions* (Albany, NY: Delmar Publishers, 1997), 5.

2. B. Schaub and R. Schaub, Alcoholics Anonymous and Psychosynthesis, in *Readings in Psychosynthesis: Theory, Process, and Practice*, vol. 2, eds. J. Weiser and T. Yeomans (Toronto: Ontario Institute for Studies in Education, 1988), 55–59.

3. Hazelden Foundation, *The Twelve Steps of Alcoholics Anonymous* (New York: Harper/ Hazelden, 1987), 2.

C H A P T E R 3 0

Incest and Child Sexual Abuse Counseling*

Nurse Healer Objective

- Explore each step of the holistic caring process when using incest or child sexual abuse interventions with various clients to facilitate the healing process.

Definitions

Child Sexual Abuse: Exploitive psychosexual activity that goes beyond the developmental level of the child, to which the child is unable to give informed consent, and that violates social taboos regarding roles and relationships.[1]

Dissociation: The experience of one's mind temporarily splitting off from one's body—a feeling of separation from the body.[2]

Flashback: A nonpsychotic episode in the present in which the person actually relives the abuse as it originally happened.

Grounding: Staying oriented in the present, rather than being engulfed by memory.

Incest: Any type of exploitive sexual experience between relatives (or surrogate relatives) before the person is eighteen years old.[3]

* Condensed from: E.J. Martin, Incest and Child Sexual Abuse Counseling, in *Holistic Nursing: A Handbook for Practice*, 4th ed., eds. B.M. Dossey, L. Keegan, C.E. Guzzetta (Sudbury, MA: Jones and Bartlett Publishers, 2005), 813–826.

Trigger: Any sight, sound, smell, or other sensory experience that stimulates recall of a memory.

Violence: A component of all incest/child sexual abuse, regardless of the intent of the perpetrator.

Holistic Caring Process

Assessment

- be personally comfortable with discussions of incest and child sexual abuse and aware of their attitudes toward it
- be aware of their personal history regarding incest and child sexual abuse
- increase their knowledge base about this problem

Nurses must then

- take responsibility for asking about incest and child sexual abuse as part of their routine nursing history-taking
- use good communication techniques
- allow time for the client to tell his or her story
- provide psychological support during the interview

Nurses also should assess

- the client's history of dissociative behaviors, which may be manifested by flashbacks, sleep disorders, and splitting or multiple personality
- the client's present level of safety, as well as the current period of safety (i.e., how long since the last abuse?)[4]

Patterns/Challenges/Needs

The following are the patterns/challenges/needs compatible with the interventions for incest and child sexual abuse survivors that are related to the 13 domains of Taxonomy II (see Chapter 14):

- Social isolation
- Impaired social interaction

- Ineffective parenting
- Sexual dysfunction
- Altered spiritual state
- Altered participation in family
- Impaired adjustment
- Ineffective coping
- Altered self-concept
- Disturbance in body concept
- Disturbance in self-esteem
- Disturbance in self-identity
- Powerlessness
- Pain
- Grief
- Anxiety
- Fear
- Post-traumatic response
- Sleep disturbance
- Self-care deficit

Outcomes

Exhibit 30–1 guides the nurse in outcomes, nursing prescriptions, and evaluation of selected incest and child sexual abuse interventions.

Therapeutic Care Plan and Implementation

BEFORE THE SESSION

- If it is the first session, prepare to be open and receptive.
- If it is not the first session, prepare by reviewing your records, reminding yourself of the "homework" asked of the client, and the goals for the present session.
- Be sure the environment is comfortable and therapeutic.
- Take time to center yourself.

AT THE BEGINNING OF THE SESSION

- After appropriate introductions or greetings, be still and listen to the client.

Exhibit 30-1 Nursing Interventions: Incest and Child Sexual Abuse

Client Outcomes	Nursing Prescriptions	Evaluation
The client will attend a social activity three times a week.	Help the client identify feelings of being socially isolated and find ways to move out of social isolation through relating to others; assist the client to choose activities in which he or she can engage comfortably.	The client reports attending social activities of his or her choosing and is comfortable in those social situations.
The client will be comfortable with altered participation in the family of origin.	Help the client understand that altered relationships with the family of origin are a common outcome when incest/child sexual abuse has occurred. Support the client in defining the parameters of relating that are within his or her sphere of comfort.	The client is able to set limits and define the level of relating with the family of origin that supports comfort and healing. This is a recurrent dynamic and will require ongoing support from and teaching by the nurse.

The client will no longer feel powerless.	Help the client identify the goal of empowerment, and support the client in the belief that he or she has the right to make decisions about his or her life.	The client reports that he or she has the right to make decisions about his or her own life.
	Support and facilitate disclosure at the client's level of comfort.	The client discloses the past trauma.
	Provide psychologic support and teach, as appropriate, principles of normal physiology and child development.	The client reports feelings of support and now understands that the body responses felt during the incest/child sexual abuse are "normal physiologic responses" and not evidence of "bad" behavior.
	Explore new behaviors, and teach those of interest to the client.	The client reports attending assertiveness training at the local YMCA.

- Support the client nonverbally and nonintrusively.
- Keep your questioning to a minimum until the client has the time needed to speak.
- Assess the verbal and nonverbal behavior of the client.

DURING THE SESSION

- Using the assessment data, validate your impressions with the client.
- Identify both the strategies that have worked well and those that have not.
- Explore these strategies with the client to gain an understanding of the outcomes.
- Hear the client's suggestions for next steps or new directions.
- Work with the client to develop a plan, including goals and interventions to achieve the desired outcomes.

AT THE END OF THE SESSION

- Summarize the session.
- Have the client validate or modify the summary.
- Assign "homework," gaining the client's agreement.
- Provide a copy of the plan for the client.
- Schedule the next session.

Specific Interventions

Nurses do not need to be experts in working with survivors to be helpful. Many helping techniques decrease the guilt and the shame associated with the long-kept "dirty" secret.

EMPOWERMENT

The client goals and outcomes are a result of a joint planning effort, and the treatment plan builds on the client's strengths. Disclosure is the first step for the survivor, but the client must feel that he or she has the nurse's permission to "tell the story."

Thus, the nurse facilitates the disclosure whenever and however the client chooses.

GROUNDING SKILLS

Many clients have developed their own ways of staying in the present, and the nurse may observe grounding behaviors during the history taking. (For example, clients may consistently touch a piece of jewelry or hold a small object in their hand.) The nurse should teach clients to assess and monitor their current level of awareness in order for them to stay grounded in the present. Grounding is especially helpful when clients experience flashbacks or dissociate. The first step is to teach survivors to identify and verbalize when they are having a flashback.

RELAXATION

Survivors of abuse often find that relaxation exercises reduce anxiety, promote grounding, and discourage dissociation. If progressive relaxation is joined with systematic desensitization, the survivor can gain some comfort in regard to anxiety-inducing people or events. (See Chapter 21 for in-depth relaxation strategies.)

WRITING

Clients can be encouraged to use various writing techniques such as journaling, writing a detailed autobiography, developing a detailed lifeline, and writing letters, even if they choose not to send them.

ANGER EXPRESSION AND MANAGEMENT

It is essential for the nurse to teach survivors first to recognize their anger, and then to express and manage it in appropriate ways. When the survivor begins to get in touch with his or her anger, it is the ideal time in treatment to explore appropriate anger management techniques. It is helpful for the survivor to learn to "dose anger" (i.e., express it in small, manageable amounts). Physical exercise also can reduce anger.

IMAGERY

An effective guided imagery technique can help a survivor remember experiences from the past and connect with the lost emotions associated with the abuse. (See Chapter 22 for more information on imagery.)

Evaluation

With the client, the nurse determines whether the client outcomes for incest and child sexual abuse (see Exhibit 30–1) were achieved. To evaluate the session further, the nurse may explore the subjective effects of the experience with the client (Exhibit 30–2).

Exhibit 30-2 Evaluating the Client's Subjective Experience of Sexual Abuse Interventions

1. Was this the first time you have ever disclosed the abuse?
2. Can you describe what you felt like before you began to disclose?
3. Did you experience physical or emotional sensations during the disclosure? Can you describe them?
4. Were you able to stay grounded during the disclosure? If not, do you know what triggered your dissociation?
5. Did you feel safe during the disclosure?
6. What did you feel immediately following the disclosure?
7. Would you be willing to disclose to another person at another time?

8. What could I have done to be more helpful to you during the disclosure?

9. Is there anything I can do right now to be helpful?

10. What is your next step or plan to integrate this disclosure experience?

Source: Data from E. Jane Martin and L. Gooding Kolkmeier, Sexual Abuse: Healing the Wounds, in *Holistic Nursing: A Handbook for Practice,* eds. B.M. Dossey et al., p. 423, © 1995, Aspen Publishers, Inc.

Nurse Healer Reflections

- Am I comfortable treating clients when sexual abuse and violence are the concerns?
- Do the interventions I use with clients work for me?

Notes

1. L.G. Kolkmeier, Sexual Abuse: Healing the Wounds, in *Holistic Nursing: A Handbook for Practice,* 2nd ed., eds. B.M. Dossey et al. (Gaithersburg, MD: Aspen Publishers, 1995), 404.

2. C. Courtois, *Healing the Incest Wound: Adult Survivors in Therapy* (New York: W.W. Norton & Co., 1988), 154.

3. J.C. Urbanic, Intrafamilial Sexual Abuse, in *Nursing Care of Survivors of Family Violence,* eds. J. Campbell and J. Humphreys (St. Louis, Mosby, 1993), 133.

4. Kolkmeier, Sexual Abuse, 407–408.

Aromatherapy—Healing Through the Senses*

Nurse Healer Objective

- Explore each step of the holistic caring process when considering healing through the senses.

Definitions

Aromatherapy: the use of essential oils for therapeutic purposes.

Clinical Aromatherapy: the use of essential oils for specific, measurable outcomes.

Chemotype: a cloned variety of a plant that always has the same chemistry as the original plant.

Essential Oil: the distillate from an aromatic plant, or the oil expressed from the peel of a citrus fruit.

The 'm' Technique®: a form of structured touch that is suitable when massage is inappropriate, either because the receiver is too fragile or the giver is not trained in massage.

The Limbic System: the oldest part of the brain; it contains the amygdala, hippocampus, thalamus, and hypothalamus.

---

* Condensed from: J. Buckle, Aromatherapy—Healing Through the Senses, in *Holistic Nursing: A Handbook for Practice*, 4th ed., eds. B.M. Dossey, L. Keegan, C.E. Guzzetta (Sudbury, MA: Jones and Bartlett Publishers, 2005), 829–851.

Learned Memory: the ability of the mind to condition the response to an aroma based on previous experience.

Methods of Application

Essential oils can be absorbed by the body in one of four ways. The methods of using essential oils that are congruent with holistic nursing practice, include inhalation, topical application, vaginal insertion, and ingestion.

Holistic Caring Process

Assessment

In preparing to use essential oils clinically, the nurses assesses the following parameters:

- the client's like or dislike of particular aromas, as this will impact the choice of essential oils
- the client's like or dislike of touch, as this will impact what method is chosen
- the client's perception of the problem, as this will indicate the targeted outcome
- the client's level of stress, as this will directly affect the oils chosen
- the client's understanding of what aromatherapy is, as this will indicate if they are expecting cure or care
- the client's skin integrity, as certain essential oils are safest to poor skin integrity
- the client's age—very young or elderly client's will need low percentages of essential oils
- the client's medical history, as previous illness could be related to the current problem
- the client's current medical status, as this will indicate which essential oils are safest to use
- the client's sleep pattern, as this will indicate if this is one of the main areas for improvement

- the client's weight and height, as these will indicate the amount of essential oil required
- the client's blood pressure, as this will indicate if hypotensive or hypertensive essential oils could be used
- the client's medication, as certain medications could be affected by essential oils
- the client's respiratory pattern, as this will indicate if there is COPD or asthma, which will indicate the method required
- the client's reproductive status, as this will indicate if the patient is pregnant, reducing the choice of essential oils
- the client's allergy status, particularly to ragweed or herbal teas, as certain essential oils would then need to be disallowed
- the client's close proximity to others who may be affected by the aromas, as this will impact which essential oils are chosen

Patterns/Challenges/Needs

The following are the patterns/challenges/needs compatible with aromatherapy that are related to the 13 domains of Taxonomy II (see Chapter 14):

- Altered circulation
- Risk of Infection
- Constipation
- Perceived constipation
- Risk for constipation
- Altered tissue perfusion (peripheral)
- Ineffective breathing pattern
- Dysfunctional ventilatory weaning Response
- Impaired tissue integrity
- Risk for impaired skin integrity
- Energy field disturbance
- Impaired verbal communication
- Social isolation
- Risk for loneliness
- Sexual dysfunction
- Caregiver role strain
- Ineffectual individual coping
- Defensive coping

- Ineffective family coping
- Family coping: potential for growth
- Decisional conflict
- Impaired physical mobility
- Impaired bed mobility
- Activity intolerance
- Fatigue
- Sleep pattern disturbance
- Delayed surgical recovery
- Adult failure to thrive
- Ineffective breastfeeding
- Bathing/hygiene self-care deficit

- Relocation stress syndrome
- Body image disturbance
- Chronic low self-esteem
- Sensory/perception/ alterations: olfactory, tactile
- Hopelessness
- Powerlessness
- Chronic confusion
- Impaired memory
- Chronic pain
- Nausea
- Dysfunctional grieving
- Chronic sorrow
- Post-trauma response
- Anxiety
- Fear

Outcomes

Exhibit 31–1 guides the nurse in outcomes, nursing prescriptions, and evaluation of selected aromatherapy intervention.

Setting Goals

It is important to establish mutually acceptable goals prior to beginning an aromatherapy and 'm' technique® session. These outcomes may be immediate or long-term, but should be relevant to aromatherapy and the role of holistic nursing care. Clients are more likely to be content with the outcomes if they are perceived to be achievable within a specified time-frame, and are deemed successful with recognizable tools such

Exhibit 31-1 Nursing Interventions: Aromatherapy

Client Outcomes	Nursing Prescriptions	Evaluation
The client will select aromas from a selection offered by the nurse.	Provide the client with various aromas to choose from that are suitable for client's condition.	The client chose aromas from a selection offered by the nurse.
The client will demonstrate positive physiologic outcomes in response to the aromatherapy and the 'm' technique® sessions, such as:	Assess the client's physiologic outcomes in response to aroma therapy and the 'm' technique® before and immediately after each session.	The client demonstrated:
• decreased respiratory rate	Evaluate the client's:	• decreased respiratory rate
• decreased heart rate	• decreased respiratory rate	• decreased heart rate
• decreased blood pressure	• decreased heart rate	• decreased blood pressure
• decreased muscle tension	• decreased blood pressure	• decreased muscle tension
• decreased fatigue	• decreased muscle tension	• decreased fatigue
• decreased pain	• decreased fatigue	• decreased pain
• improved physical mobility	• decreased pain	• improved physical mobility
• improved bed mobility		• improved bed mobility
		• improved activity tolerance
		• improved sleep pattern
		• improved surgical recovery
		• improved ability to thrive
		(continues)

Exhibit 31-1   (continued)

Client Outcomes	Nursing Prescriptions	Evaluation
• improved activity tolerance • improved sleep pattern • improved surgical recovery • improved ability to thrive • improved breastfeeding • improved self-care • reduced nausea • reduced constipation • reduced risk of infection The client will demonstrate positive psychologic outcomes in response to the aromatherapy and the 'm' technique® sessions such as: • improved body image • improved self-esteem	• improved physical mobility • improved bed mobility • improved activity tolerance • improved sleep pattern • improved surgical recovery • improved ability to thrive • improved breastfeeding • improved self-care • reduced nausea • reduced constipation • reduced risk of infection Assess the client's psychologic outcomes in response to aroma therapy and the 'm' technique® before and immediately after each session. Evaluate the client's:	• improved breastfeeding • improved self-care • reduced nausea • reduced constipation • reduced risk of infection The client demonstrated: • improved body image • improved self-esteem • improved olfactory ability • improved tactile ability • reduced hopelessness • reduced powerlessness

- improved olfactory ability
- improved tactile ability
- reduced hopelessness
- reduced powerlessness
- reduced confusion
- improved memory
- more functional grieving
- reduced sorrow
- improved trauma response
- reduced anxiety
- reduced fear
- more effective coping
- less decisional conflict
- better family coping

- improved body image
- improved self-esteem
- improved olfactory ability
- improved tactile ability
- reduced hopelessness
- reduced powerlessness
- reduced confusion
- improved memory
- more functional grieving
- reduced sorrow
- improved trauma response
- reduced anxiety
- reduced fear
- more effective coping
- less decisional conflict
- better family coping

- reduced confusion
- improved memory
- more functional grieving
- reduced sorrow
- improved trauma response
- reduced anxiety
- reduced fear
- more effective coping
- less decisional conflict
- better family coping

as visual analogs. It is recommended that such goals are judged by using a visual analog scale (0–10), where 0 is lack of the symptom (such as pain) and 10 is the worst imaginable symptom (such as pain). Informed consent (with written consent where possible) is required before using essential oils.

Therapeutic Care Plan and Implementation

BEFORE THE SESSION

- If in a clinical area, inform other people that aromatherapy will be used and assess if they are comfortable with the aromas that will be used.
- Request no interruptions for the period required. This could be 5 minutes for a hand 'm' technique® using essential oils, or 15 minutes for hand, face, and feet. Allow 15 minutes for inhalation.
- Discuss the length of the session, the required outcome, and the method to be used.
- Ask client to empty the bladder for comfort.
- Prepare the hospital bed or surface on which you will be working. Adjust the bed height for your convenience.
- Ensure the temperature of the room is appropriate.
- Ask the client to remove eyeglasses if using direct inhalation as a method.
- Prepare the environment for optimal relaxation if this is the purpose of the session.
- Place a clean towel under the hand or foot for 'm' technique®.
- Wash hands.
- Prepare mixture of essential oils in carrier oil if being applied topically to the skin.
- Prepare diffuser with mixture of undiluted essential oils if inhalation is being used.
- Prepare compress with either water or carrier oil for wound care.

- Prepare bath for emersion of limb or body.
- Prepare basin with very hot water for steam inhalation.
- Prepare basin with warm water and essential oils for body wash.
- Focus on your healing intention and then begin.

AT THE BEGINNING OF THE SESSION

- Tell the client what you are going to do before you do it.
- Tell the client which part of the body you are going to touch before you touch it.
- Make sure that the limb is supported.
- Ask the client to tell you what the pressure feels like to them (on a level of 0–10) if you are using the 'm' technique®.
- Warm your hands by rubbing them together.
- Apply a small amount of dilute essential oil in to one hand if using the 'm' technique®.
- Put required drops of essential oil in basin for steam inhalation.
- Put required number of drops of essential oil in diffuser.
- Begin slowly and rhythmically if using the 'm' technique®.
- Help position client above steaming bowl for inhalation and place towel over head and shoulders.
- Begin applying dilute essential oils to wound or burn.

DURING THE SESSION

- Maintain constant pressure, rhythm, and speed if using manual therapy.
- Discourage conversation.
- Encourage client to focus on the treatment.
- If client is using inhalation method encourage them to breath deeply.
- Have tissues available for expectoration if steam inhalation is used.

- Have empty basin available if essential oil is being used for nausea.
- Stay with a confused, elderly, infirm, or very young patient if inhalation or bath is being used.
- Reassess the client as you move through the session.

AT THE END OF THE SESSION

- Remove any apparatus used for aromatherapy (basin, bath, diffuser).
- If the client has gone to sleep gently wake him/her after a few moments.
- Tell the client that you have finished the session.
- Dry skin if bath has been used.

Specific Interventions

- Have the client identify and verbalize any changes or experiences that occurred during the session.
- The nurse may reassess physical parameters such as blood pressure, pulse, and respiration.
- The nurse may suggest that the treatment is self-applied at regular intervals.
- The nurse may make up a series of treatments in a bottle for such self-application.
- The nurse may schedule a follow-up treatment.

Nurse Healer Reflections

- What is important for me to know before I begin using essential oils?
- How do I know whether to apply an essential oil topically or inhale it?
- What is my experience of inhaling the five essential oils in this chapter?
- What is my experience of applying the five essential oils topically to my skin at 5%?

CHAPTER 32

Relationship-Centered Care and Healing Initiative in a Community Hospital*

Nurse Healer Objective

- Explore the components of relationship-centered care and a healing initiative in a community hospital.

Definitions

Healing Health Care: an applied philosophy that facilitates and promotes healing of the "whole person"—body, mind, and spirit. It responds to and serves the unique needs of individuals, groups, organizations, communities, and cultures. A healing health care project demonstrates the ethic of healing health care: healing ourselves, our relationships, and our communities.

The Association of Healing Health Care Projects: The mission of the Association of Healing Health Care Projects is to both inspire and support health care models that exemplify human caring and healing.

About St. Charles

In 1990, St. Charles, like many hospitals, was in the process of restructuring services in an effort to prepare for a rapidly

* Condensed from: N. Moore, Relationship-Centered Care and Healing Initiative in a Community Hospital in *Holistic Nursing: A Handbook for Practice*, 4th ed., eds. B.M. Dossey, L. Keegan, C.E. Guzzetta (Sudbury, MA: Jones and Bartlett Publishers, 2005), 857–882.

changing health care environment. The Healing Health Care Philosophy was developed to guide the hospital in intentionally preserving and enhancing its mission during the chaotic change.[1] This included how to integrate relationship-centered care and to achieve healthy relationships among practitioners, patients and the community.[2]

In 2000, St. Charles Medical Center was honored with the Norman Cousin's Award for relationship-centered care.

Healing Ourselves and Our Relationships

Early in the Healing Health Care Philosophy implementation we believed that we needed to create something tangible, so that people could understand the philosophy. It eventually became crystal clear that the essence of healing is in our relationships. As a result, we developed personal growth and development workshops, *People-Centered Teams: Healing Our Workplace I*. All employees now attend the workshops as part of orientation, and the workshops are open to the community, as well as employees that wish to retake them. Healing Health Care coaches are available to assist staff with the integration of the newly learned skills, and all teams set expectations and use the skills they've acquired by developing written team agreements that are integral to each team's functioning. In recognition of the increasingly stressful work environment, we also have added a second workshop, *Resiliency and Renewal*, in collaboration with Adaptive Learning Systems.

Other resources to support healing ourselves and our relationships include a Caregiver Assistance Program (CAP) and critical incident stress debriefings. CAP offers on-site confidential counseling that is available to caregivers and their family members, as well as assessment and referral to appropriate resources. The critical incident stress debriefings are available through social services for teams or individuals experiencing unusual amounts of stress, such as caring for many critical patients for a prolonged period of time or helping in a severe accident.

Patient-Focused and Family-Focused Care

The most effective way to promote healing is for patients to become actively involved in their care. Patient-focused and family-focused care actively involves patients and family members or significant others as the patient desires in the care process and provides services based on their needs.

A major source of nurse burnout is that nurses often work on their assumptions of what the patient needs. This can lead to dissatisfied patients as well as burned-out nurses. Prioritizing care based on the patient's needs as identified by the patient is one of the most important nursing skills. We now are using, as a consistent service standard, Sharon K. Dingman's *The Caring Model*™ that consists of five behaviors that are part of an organization-wide or nursing department change initiative that are as follows:[3]

1. Introduce yourself to patients and explain your role in their care/service today.
2. Call the patient by his/her preferred name.
3. *Direct caregivers*, sit at the bedside for at least five minutes each shift to plan and review the patient's care and outcomes.
   Nondirect caregivers, sit if possible, to discuss procedures, processes, and services involved in attaining desired outcomes.
4. Use touch, handshake, or touch on the arm.
5. Use the mission, vision, and values statements in planning patient care.

Nurses themselves are the most important therapeutic intervention. We are people caring for people. We use technology, but it usually is as an extension of ourselves. The need for enhanced anxiety and pain management, led to the development of *Pain/Anxiety Management: Integrating Healing Health Care Principles Core Competencies*.

Life Skills

To educate patients advising them of health risks and what they can do about them became the Center for Health and Learning (CHL, or Center). The CHL, funded primarily from community and caregiver donations, is now at the front door of St. Charles Medical Center.

The Center's signature lifestyle-change programs (*New Directions*, a ten-week behavior change program; *Health Coach Services*; and a one-day *Life Choice Seminar*) incorporate a body-mind-spirit approach to making and sustaining lifestyle and behavior changes in support of optimal wellness that defines the components necessary to support successful lifestyle change.

New Directions Program

New Directions is a ten-week program designed to assist patients with symptoms of chronic disease and stress. Using an integrated model of cognitive behavior change, and standard medical care, this body-mind-spirit program is supporting people in making life changes and experiencing greater health.

Health Coach Services

Health Coach Services provide one-on-one support to individuals by a Health Coach Nurse in all aspects of their health care: reducing risk factors for heart disease, diabetes, and cancer; managing stress; preparing for surgery; and overall lifestyle changes. The Health Coach Nurses assist people in overcoming barriers to physical, emotional, and spiritual health through better managing stress and creating more balance in their lives. Each participant creates a health action plan.

Life-Death Transition

St. Charles is committed to the continual development of the skills and presence necessary to assist dying patients and their families. Oregon passed the nation's first physician-assisted suicide legislation. The SCMC Board of Directors viewed this act by the people of Oregon as a message that health care, in general, has failed in supporting people through the dying process. As a result, the Board directed the hospital staff to improve end-of-life care.

The team developed an education plan, policies and procedures, and preprinted orders, and consistently works to support physicians and caregivers in caring for their patients in the dying process. A Comfort Care Patient Checklist was developed and implemented.

The Deschutes County Coalition for Quality End-of-Life Care

The second track for improving end-of-life care, the Deschutes County Coalition for Quality End-of-Life Care, focuses beyond the walls of the hospital to the community and all of the various settings where people die.

Arts in the Hospital

Curing is of the body. Caring is of the soul. The arts speak to the soul. The environment is a mirror of the individual and of the culture. It echoes the values of the culture. Art enriches the environment and can connect people to purpose and meaning by representing the organization's unique mythology. The St. Charles Arts in the Hospital program includes art, music, and humor (see Resources.) Healing Health care for information on C.A.R.E. (continuous ambient relaxation environment) audiovisual system to be used as a TV channel.

Healing Our Community

In 1995, Jim Lussier, CEO, formed the Central Oregon Health Council (COHC) as a resource for accomplishing our mission. The council now has 35 member agencies, including such agencies as the Bend/Lapine School District, the Commission on Children and Families, the City of Bend, and the Central Oregon Council on Aging.

The Council developed a mission statement, community health values, and benchmarks for measurement. The Council focuses on five methods of creating a healthy community:

- Public education focusing on health
- Developing new public–private partnerships
- Resource development and alignment
- Monitoring progress of benchmarks and reporting to the community
- Influencing public policy

Principle-Based Care Model

The Healing Health Care Philosophy, along with the collective vision of both management and staff nurses, guided the recent revision of the system's care model, the health management model. The health management model is principle-based, relationship-centered, resource-based, and outcome-focused. The person accesses care through prevention, wellness, and/or intervention services. Prevention and wellness services are provided through the Center for Health and Learning. Intervention services (inpatient and outpatient) are provided through physicians and primary nursing. The primary nurse is responsible for developing a therapeutic relationship and a plan of care throughout the patient's stay on his or her unit. The primary nurse works as part of a team with either a licensed practical nurse (LPN) or a certified nursing assistant (CNA), along with physicians, case managers, and other disciplines as needed. The plan of care is respected and followed by the entire health care team. When patients are discharged, they are connected to the appropriate services of the Center for Health and Learning, as well as other community resources as needed.

Nurse Healer Reflections

- How does the environment affect my own healing?
- After reflecting on a recent time when I felt most helpful to a patient, what do I think contributed to this experience? Ask myself why at least five times.
- What can I do now in my work environment to better support healing?
- What does the ethic of the Healing Health Care Philosophy—healing ourselves, our relationships, and our communities—mean to me personally?

Notes

1. N. Moore, Relationship-Centered Service: St. Charles Medical Center and Perspective: How You Can Become Involved, in *Integrating Complementary Medicine Into Health Systems*, ed. N. Faass (Gaithersburg, MD: Aspen Publishers, 2001).
2. C.P. Tresolini and the Pew-Fetzer Task Force, *Health Professions and Relationship-Centered Care* (San Francisco, CA: Pew Health Professions Commission, 1994).
3. S. Dingman, M. Williams, D. Fosbinder, and M. Warnick, Implementing a Caring Model to Improve Patient Satisfaction, *Journal of Nursing Administration* 29, no. 12 (1999):30–37.

Resources

St. Charles Medical Center, Bend, Oregon
Phone: 541-385-6390
www.scmc.org/chm.htlm

Healing HealthCare Systems: *www.healing health.com*; email: healhealth@aol.com

The Creative Connection:
email: creativeconnection @oakweb.com

Society for The Arts in Healthcare:
www.thesah.org

Symposium on Health Care Design:
www.hcaredesign.com

Planetree: *www.planetree.org*

Creative HealthCare Management: *www.chcm.com*

IMPAQ: *www.impaqcorp.com*

CHAPTER 33

Exploring Integrative Medicine and the Healing Environment: The Story of a Large Urban Acute Care Hospital*

Nurse Healer Objective

- Explore the components of integrative medicine and the healing environment in a large urban acute care hospital.

Definitions

Total Healing Environment: a health care environment that demonstrates aspects of healing in the physical space, relationships, therapeutic interventions, and leadership.

Integrative Medicine(IM): a philosophy of health care practice that emphasizes the 'whole person' view of health and healing and, in practice, blends conventional, alternative, and complementary interventions to optimize curing and healing.

* Condensed from: L. Knutson, Exploring Integrative Medicine and the Healing Environment: The Story of a Large Urban Acute Care Hospital, in *Holistic Nursing: A Handbook for Practice*, 4th ed., eds. B.M. Dossey, L. Keegan, C.E. Guzzetta (Sudbury, MA: Jones and Bartlett Publishers, 2005), 885–898.

289

Quality Initiatives: processes that utilize specialties of clinical practice in therapeutic partnerships to create improved patient care.

Holistic Nurse Clinician: a certified Holistic Nurse who performs needs assessments of patients and the clinical environment and initiates appropriate healing interventions to enable positive changes in health.

Total Healing Environment Model: Large Urban Acute Care Hospital

Abbott Northwestern Hospital is the largest not-for-profit hospital in the Minneapolis area. Each year, the hospital provides comprehensive health care for more than 200,000 patients and their families from the Twin Cities area and throughout the upper midwest. More than 5000 nonmedical employees, 1600 physicians, 2000 nurses, and 550 volunteers work as a team for the benefit of each patient served. Abbott Northwestern Hospital is a part of Allina Hospitals & Clinics, a family of hospitals, clinics, and care services in Minnesota and Western Wisconsin. Abbott Northwestern Hospital's services include:

- complete medical, surgical, and critical care for patients age 12 and older
- 24-hour emergency services
- multispecialty care and clinical expertise in behavioral health services, cardiovascular services, medical/surgical services, neuroscience, oncology, orthopedics, rehabilitation, spine care, and women's health
- outpatient care in more than 50 different specialty areas
- innovative and individual pain treatment
- overnight guest accommodations for patients' families and friends, and for outpatients
- education programs, support services, and public health screenings
- outreach programs to improve the health of the community

The concept for the Healing Environment at Abbott Northwestern Hospital, which was introduced in 2000, stemmed from the recognition of the needs of the patients, their families, and the staff. This recognition came from key nursing leaders, the CEO, the hospital's Board, and significant philanthropic donors. This partnership gave energy to the driving force in determining the desired culture change and holistic approach to care delivery. It was key nursing leaders in collaboration with executive leadership that earmarked the framework for the Total Healing Environment.

There are four primary components to Abbott Northwestern Hospital's concept of a total healing environment:

EXTERNAL/PHYSICAL

The external/physical elements of the Total Healing Environment are related to the visible and concrete. These include the appearance and privacy of the patient rooms, as well as the appearance of the public spaces, the views from the windows, the quality of the air, and environmental sounds.

EXTERNAL/PSYCHOLOGICAL

The external/psychological elements refer to how staff relate to one another and to patients and their families; the customers' perspectives of the hospital reputation; the expertise of staff; the quality, variety, and efficiency of services; inclusion of the patient and family in all aspects of care; and access to information.

INTERNAL/PHYSICAL

The internal/physical elements address the ability to treat and cure disease, manage physical pain, and optimize the body's health.

INTERNAL/PSYCHOLOGICAL

The internal/psychological elements emphasize supporting positive mental and spiritual well-being, and promoting self-responsibility and acceptance, and are sensitive to individual beliefs and values related to health and healing.

Integrative Medicine

Integrative medicine is a comprehensive, primary care system that emphasizes wellness and healing of the whole person (bio-psycho-socio-spiritual dimensions) as major goals, above and beyond suppression of a specific somatic disease.[1] Integrative Medicine is not CAM (Complementary and Alternative Medicine). Integrative medicine is patient-centered, healing-oriented care that emphasizes the patient–caregiver relationship. It focuses on the least invasive, least toxic, and least costly methods to promote health by blending the practices of CAM and conventional, Western medicine. Central to integrative medicine is the view of the whole person as a dynamic being interrelating with his or her environment, both internal and external, and that this interrelationship is the key to health and well-being.[2]

Integrative Medicine Team

The Integrative Medicine Team is composed of six members:

Medical Director. Overall accountability, physician relationships, philanthropic initiatives, national trending, external partnerships.

Director of Programs and Services. Strategic plan and financial accountability, personnel and HR activities, performance improvement, stakeholder relationships, executive leadership for patient care communities, partner with nursing leadership.

Holistic Nurse Clinician (HNC [certification through the American Holistic Nurses Certification Corporation (AHNCC)]).[3] Provides integrative medicine patient consultations, participates in program development, staff education and training, facilitates and manages the continuum of care, partners in research and quality initiatives.

Healing Coach. Patient advocate; provides emotional support through the continuum of care, participates in the "Healing Plan of Care."

Education and Research Coordinator. Provides resources for IM education, plans and implements clinical research and quality initiatives.

IM Practitioners. Provide specific alternative and complementary services; practitioners employed have a primary specialty service (i.e., massage therapy) but are trained to provide other services (guided imagery, healing touch) as well.

Integrative Medicine Components
- Relationship-Centered Care
- Partnerships
- Whole person view
- Focus is on healing
- Emphasis on self-responsibility
- Prevention
- Blending of conventional and nonconventional health care practices

Conclusions

We are in unprecedented times in the delivery of health care by hospitals. Patients, practitioners, and hospital leadership are recognizing the need to engage in an integrative approach to health and healing. This approach requires that hospitals invest in people as their bottom line in an effort to optimize the hospital experience for the patient. A healing environment begins by acknowledging that the current hospital environment emphasizes curing and is devoid of healing both for the patient and the employee.

Nurse Healer Reflections

- How do I contribute to the healing environment of a hospital?
- How can I cultivate the knowledge, skills, and intuition in the manifestation of professional healing relationships?

Notes

1. I.R. Bell et al., Integrative Medicine and Systemic Outcomes Research, Issues in the Emergence of a New Model for Primary Health Care, *Archives of Internal Medicine* 162 (2002):133–140.
2. R. Snyderman and A. Weil, Integrative Medicine: Bringing Medicine Back to Its Roots, *Archives of Internal Medicine* 162 (2002):395–397.
3. American Holistic Nurses' Certification Corporation (AHNCC). email: ahncc@flash.net.

INDEX

A

Abbott Northwestern Hospital, 290–294

accounting of self, 79
emotional intelligence, 209
holistic self-assessments, 115–120
life review, 139
self-reflection, 131–140

acculturation, defined, 95

active listening. *See* listening

acupressure, 197, 206

acute pain, 42–44. *See also* pain
assessment imagery, 183–184

addiction, defined, 251

addiction and recovery counseling, 251–259
smoking cessation, 241–248

advanced standards for holistic nursing, 8

aerobic exercise, defined, 151

aesthetic knowing, 18
cocreative process, 19–20

affirmations (self-talk), 120, 231
denial, defined, 251
empowerment, 266
negative self-talk, 237
smoking cessation, 247

AHNA (American Holistic Nurses' Association)
address and contact information, 11
Description of Holistic Nursing, 26–27
person, defining, 28–30
standards and certification, 7–8

alcoholism counseling, 251–259

allopathic therapies, 3, 8–10
integrative medicine (IM), 289–294

alternative therapies, 9–10. *See also* CAM therapies
integrative medicine (IM), 289–294

ambience, defined, 83

American Holistic Nurses' Association. *See* AHNA

amygdala, 40–41

anaerobic exercise, defined, 151

anger expression and management, 267
dying and, 222

anthropocentrism, defined, 83

antioxidants, defined, 141

archetype, defined, 209

art of holistic nursing, 17–22

arts, 285
creating, as act of self-reflection, 137
expressive. *See* communication; relationships